Irritable Bladder
& Incontinence

A NATURAL APPROACH

Jennifer Hunt

Irritable Bladder
& Incontinence

A NATURAL APPROACH

Jennifer Hunt

Ulysses Press Berkeley, CA
1998

This book has been written and published strictly for informational purposes, and in no way should it be used as a substitute for consultation with your medical doctor or health care professional. All facts in this book came from medical files, clinical journals, scientific publications, personal interviews, published trade books, self-published materials by experts, magazine articles, and the personal-practice experiences of the authorities quoted or sources cited. You should not consider educational material herein to be the practice of medicine or to replace consultation with a physician or other medical practitioner. The author and publisher are providing you with information in this work so that you can have the knowledge and can choose, at your own risk, to act on that knowledge. The author and publisher also urge all readers to be aware of their health status and to consult health professionals before beginning any health program, including changes in dietary habits.

All names and identifying characteristics of real persons have been changed in the text to protect their confidentiality.

Published by: Ulysses Press
            P.O. Box 3440
            Berkeley, CA 94703-3440

Library of Congress Catalog Card Number: 97-61006

ISBN: 1-56975-089-0

First published as *Coping Successfully with Your Irritable Bladder* by Sheldon Press

Printed in Canada by Best Book Manufacturers

10 9 8 7 6 5 4 3 2 1

Editor: Mark Woodworth
Cover Design: B & L Design
Cover Illustration: Nude #3 by Diana Ong/SuperStock
Editorial and production staff: Lily Chou, Aaron Newey
Typesetter: David Wells
Indexer: Sayre Van Young

Distributed in the United States by Publishers Group West and in Canada by Raincoast Books

*This book is dedicated
to my parents,
with love.*

Acknowledgments

I wish to thank the staff of the department of urological gynecology at St. Mary's Hospital, Manchester, England, for their help, particularly Sister Jill Lord, Dr. Tony Smith and Gordon Hosker. Also all my colleagues at the department of clinical psychology at Withington Hospital, Manchester, for their encouragement, and a special thank-you to Dr. David Unwin for his advice and support.

Contents

Introduction

You may be wondering if this book is for you. You have perhaps skimmed through it and seen a couple of diagrams and looked at the table of contents page. You are not too sure if you actually *have* an "irritable bladder" and, even if you have, whether reading about it will help. So, I will start by explaining whom this book has been written for and then will go on to describe how it might help you.

If your life tends to be planned around your bladder, and if it influences your daily life, relationships and activities and how you feel, then read on. Do you feel uneasy if you don't know where the nearest restroom is? Do you try to avoid situations where a safe and clean restroom may not be within easy reach, such as traveling or going to the movies? Are you constantly aware of how full your bladder is, how much you've drunk and when you last went to the bathroom? If the answer to any of these questions is "yes," then this book was written for you.

Irritable bladder, as I will use the term, can refer to a variety of bladder problems. These range from having to empty the bladder frequently when feeling nervous (something everyone experiences to a certain extent), to bladder pain and discomfort, to incontinence. Just like irritable bowel syndrome, which you probably have heard of, there are several symptoms that you may experience. What irritable bowel syndrome and irritable bladder syndrome have in common is that medical treatments (such as drug therapy and surgery) are not always completely successful in relieving the symptoms. You may have had this experience yourself. This book contains information about common medical treatments as well as simple approaches to help you with your problem.

Bladder and bowel problems also have other things in common. The first, and most important, is that we find it enormously difficult to talk about either of them openly, even to our family physician. We try to keep them hidden from our family, friends and colleagues for fear that we will be judged harshly, and because we feel that the problem in some way reflects on our character or self-control. There is an un-spoken taboo surrounding bladder problems; this makes it difficult to discuss or understand them. This is something that is emphasized at a very early age and can make our experiences of such problems all the more upsetting and difficult to cope with. The second common factor results from our inability to discuss these problems openly; we do not realize how very common these symptoms are and what sim-ple measures we can adopt to help us overcome them. This books aims to educate you about how these problems arise and to assist you in designing your own plan to improve and cope successfully with your symptoms.

How common *are* the symptoms we're talking about? Research has shown that at least 20 percent of women have problems with fre-quency and urgency of urination. That is to say that one in every five women has difficulties, often feeling the need to urinate and having to visit the toilet a lot. I am constantly struck by the number of people who have bladder problems. When I have spoken to colleagues and friends about my interest in this area, they reveal their personal expe-riences, such as having to get out of bed at night for "one last visit" even if they have only been about 20 minutes earlier. Some of the people I have seen in the course of my daily work may have been uri-nating 20 or more times a day! Naturally, this is incredibly disruptive to everyday life.

The number of people with bladder problems is more than likely underestimated, because people are often reluctant to reveal them. Therefore, any of the figures you see quoted are probably too low. Men and women of all ages experience bladder problems, although men seem to have fewer difficulties, particularly with incontinence. For this reason, I am aiming this book primarily at women, though much of what I say applies equally to men, and I do give specific information where it is relevant.

Estimates for incontinence vary, depending on who is studied and how the questions are asked, but you may be surprised to learn that over 30 percent of the adult female population (that's one in every three) are occasionally troubled by incontinence, and over 10 percent are regularly incontinent (consider the great number of "adult diapers" you see stocked along supermarket and drugstore aisles, not all intended for the elderly or bed-bound invalids). As you can see, if you are experiencing bladder problems, you are not alone. In fact, it is practically impossible *not* to know someone with similar problems, even if you've never discussed it with them.

It is difficult to say exactly how common incontinence is, because defining the problem is not easy. Generally, it is defined as an "involuntary loss of urine." As you can imagine, there is a great deal of variation in the amount and frequency of such loss. Also, the term itself obviously has negative associations, and people are often understandably reluctant to use it. Some may prefer to say they are "damp" or that they "leak a little." I use the term "incontinence" to refer to the unwanted loss of urine and hope that any embarrassment you feel will soon be overcome. I will use the term "urinate" to describe the act of emptying the bladder voluntarily. Other terminology will be described as we go along. Please do not assume this book is not for you if you don't suffer from incontinence. The book is aimed at coping with urgency and frequency problems, which can be aspects of incontinence but are also commonly experienced without it.

Why, then, is this book necessary? And why, you might be wondering, has it been written by a psychologist? First let me explain my background. I am a clinical psychologist working with adults who have health problems. I have a particular interest in bladder difficulties and have researched this area. In my experience of working with patients with a wide variety of health difficulties, from diabetes and arthritis to headaches and heart disease, I find that it is the person's reaction to their difficulties that determines how they cope, both practically and emotionally, and this style of coping can in turn affect the course of the illness. There are no clear-cut distinctions between what is "medical" or "physical" and what is "emotional" or "psychological," even with "bodily" problems. Perhaps I should illustrate my point.

Two men, John and Tony, injure their backs in a similar way after slipping on some ice. Both are in a lot of pain. Their doctors reassure them that nothing is broken or permanently damaged and prescribe some painkillers.

John is distressed; he has important deadlines to keep at work and can't afford to take time off because he is hoping for a promotion. He was already feeling stressed and this is almost the last straw. He takes one or two more painkillers than he should and struggles off to the office. He manages in this way for two days and then is told to go home because his co-workers can see he is in pain and is not working well. He is feeling somewhat depressed about his inability to struggle on and goes to bed. The pain seems almost unbearable and he continues taking his painkillers. After two days in bed worrying about work, the pain is still bad. He calls the doctor. The doctor is surprised that John is so distressed and wonders if she has missed something in her diagnosis. She refers John to an orthopedic specialist and also prescribes stronger painkillers, thinking it will reassure John. This causes John to worry even more about his pain, thinking it could be something serious, and he continues to be concerned about work. He tries to get up, but worries about aggravating the problem, so he stays in bed. He feels that things are out of his control.

Tony is also worried. He, too, has important things to do at work. He thinks about the pros and cons of struggling on and decides it is important to take it easy for a week. He phones in sick. He stays in bed for a few days, reading and watching television to take his mind off the pain. After this, he slowly starts to do more things, resting if the pain worsens. He feels reassured that things are getting slightly better over time, and in a phone call his doctor agrees. Tony returns to work after a week and is careful not to overdo it. He feels in control, and soon things are nearly back to normal.

These stories may seem a little exaggerated, but I hope you get the idea. People's *reactions* (that is, their thoughts and feelings) influence how they cope and recover. There are many factors involved in how you react to bladder problems. If you can look at how you view things, then you are better able to change how you cope with them. Coping, or having a sense of practical and emotional control, can make an enormous difference in your daily life and can actually reduce the symptoms and distress that you—like all humans—suffer.

People with long-term bladder problems naturally feel that their bladders rule their lives. You may find that you have adapted over time by avoiding certain situations or activities, but still the problem is often on your mind. Taking a step back to look at the problem can help you cope with it more successfully.

Let me give you another, more relevant, example.

Megan had not suffered any major health problems—just a couple of painful bouts of cystitis (bladder infection) in her twenties. She is an active person who likes to do things well and often leaves herself little time to relax.

Over a period of time Megan noticed that she needed to urinate more and more often, up to 20 times a day. She would experience a strong need to urinate that went away for a while after she had voided but soon came back. In an attempt to go to the toilet less often she began to drink less fluid, thinking there would be less need to go. She worried that if she didn't urinate when she felt the first urge the discomfort would get worse or she might become "incontinent"—a word she dreaded. These worries led her to urinate whenever she could and whenever she was near a bathroom, "just in case." For example, she would always go to the bathroom two or three times before departing for work or going out. She also noticed that when she was feeling stressed or upset her bladder was even more sensitive. She worried about her bladder and what people would think of her trips to the toilet every 20 minutes (did they think she was bored with them? or forcing herself to vomit up her food? or doing something illicit?). She avoided being away from a bathroom for too long—especially avoiding long road trips and turning down vacation offers with friends—and often stayed home as a result.

After Megan was given some general information and advice about slowly reducing how often she urinates, increasing her fluid intake to encourage the bladder to work normally and practicing some relaxation techniques, she reduced her frequency of urinating to a "normal" level, and she no longer feels discomfort or worries about her bladder's ruling her life.

The aim of this book is to increase your sense of control over your particular bladder difficulties. The first step is to understand the problem: the first three chapters give you the information you need to understand the symptoms you are experiencing—what causes them and what kinds of medical tests and procedures you may encounter. Chapter 4 discusses the physical and emotional factors that can affect how your bladder works.

Chapters 5, 6 and 7 tell how you can make changes to improve your symptoms as much as possible. Since your bladder is only as healthy as the rest of you, general lifestyle and health issues are discussed in Chapter 8.

Chapters 9 and 10 are aimed at recognizing and modifying the effects that stress and worry can have on your bladder problems. Although it is common knowledge that the bladder is extremely sensitive to worry or anxiety—particularly if that anxiety is about the bladder itself—this is an area where people receive little help. You will find help here.

Summary

Millions of people have irritable bladder problems. The main problems are urgency and frequency of urination. There is enormous variety in the way people react and cope with bladder problems, and it can be particularly difficult to discuss them.

Whatever your particular problems are, this book can help you increase your knowledge about the bladder, so that you can control and improve your symptoms and cope successfully with them.

CHAPTER ONE

What Are Your Symptoms?

The very first and most important step in learning how to better cope with your bladder problems is to know exactly how things are at the moment. This may sound a little strange, because you may think you know what your difficulties are already, —but you need to be specific and clear from the start, for a number of reasons. First, this will enable you in a few weeks' or months' time to look at how things have improved, which can be a great motivator to continue making changes. Second, because the problems you are experiencing may upset you, there will be an understandable temptation to either underplay the problem ("If I ignore it, it will go away") or feel overwhelmed by it ("Things are so bad, there's nothing I can do"). Neither of these viewpoints will help you cope with nor control your symptoms in the long run. Being as objective as possible can help. Third, keeping a record of your symptoms is an essential part of planning the right program for you. And finally, if you have a good idea of what your symptoms are, you can better help the medical or holistic staffs you consult understand and treat the problem in the best way possible.

The first step is to be clear about the nature of the beast! Irritable bladder symptoms include frequent bladder emptying, feelings of urgency to urinate and sometimes discomfort. Incontinence sufferers often experience these problems to a greater or lesser extent. Urgency and frequency are by no means always linked with incontinence, although sufferers may fear this happening. For this reason, incontinence is also discussed in the book. Other symptoms can include bowel problems, abdominal aches and headaches.

Bladder symptoms are generally of three types—frequency and urgency of urination, discomfort and incontinence. Let's consider each of these in more detail and then discuss ways in which you can monitor your own symptoms.

Frequency and Urgency

Most bladder problems are accompanied by some change in the frequency of urination—how often you visit the toilet to empty your bladder. Usually there is also a change in the feeling of the bladder, which leads to a change in a person's behavior. Urgency or "urge" is a sudden, strong need to empty the bladder. If someone uses the bathroom more often, this is often because of an increased feeling in the urge to urinate. If someone uses the bathroom less often, then there may be a reduced feeling or urge to urinate.

What is normal urinary frequency? As with all human experience and functions, everyone is different. According to researchers, for most people, frequency is about six or seven times in a 24-hour period. However, anywhere between four and ten times a day can also be perfectly normal, in the sense that the person is healthy and not concerned about his or her bladder and there have been no unexplained changes.

What is normal also depends on a large number of other things that affect the bladder—for example, the amount and type of fluid you drink, the climate, how active you are, your age and your genetic makeup, to name a few. Some of these factors and others will be discussed in greater detail in Chapters 2 and 4. It is unusual, however, to have to get up more than once a night to urinate. Try to work out how often you usually urinate each day (don't worry if it seems like a lot; it's important to be honest with yourself). Do you have to get out of bed at night to empty your bladder? If so, how many times? What is it that leads to your emptying your bladder? Is it an actual urge to urinate, or do you often go out of habit or "just in case?" Start to think about this last question the next time you go.

Very frequent urination can interfere enormously with everyday life and can become a source of great worry and embarrassment. This can become a major concern, causing you to plan your life around the problem. In fact, it is usually not just the *number* of times the person has to urinate that is the main concern, but rather the uncomfortable feeling of the need and urgency to urinate, as well as the worry about the problem. Again, there is a great deal of variation both in the amount and kind of urgency or discomfort that people experience and in the range of possible causes.

Pain and Discomfort

Sometimes people's major concern about their bladder has to do with changes in localized feeling. As we all know, the feeling of urgency or need to empty the bladder can be rather uncomfortable as well as preoccupying, making it difficult to think about anything else. If you are emptying the bladder frequently, it is likely that you are also suffering some discomfort in terms of urgency. Many people find their discomfort is temporarily relieved by emptying the bladder. Is this true for you? Often people have fears about the discomfort getting worse and use bladder emptying to prevent this. Of course, this only works in the short term because over time you are training your bladder to cope with smaller volumes of urine and to become more sensitive. I will discuss this kind of vicious circle more in Chapter 4.

There are also other kinds of discomfort associated with bladder problems. Some people experience continual discomfort and aching around the groin or backaches. For some, urination itself is painful.

Do you suffer from any discomfort or pain? If so, where do you experience the feelings? What is the pattern of the discomfort? Does it come and go? If so, what makes it worse or better? Spend a few moments thinking about this.

Incontinence

As we have discussed, losing urine involuntarily is a very common problem. Yet there is enormous variation when it comes to people's experiences of incontinence. I would certainly defy any woman to say that she has never laughed or coughed so hard that she has wet herself! I will describe how and why this occurs in the next chapter.

At the other end of the spectrum, a person may have to deal with being continually wet or with losing a large amount of urine at one time. The *pattern* of urine loss is important when determining the kind of problem you have and how to treat it. Begin to consider your own individual pattern.

If you lose urine, is it linked with particular events, such as coughing, or with certain movements, such as riding your bicycle vigorously? Is it worse when you are feeling stressed? How many times a day/week is it happening? Does it follow a strong and sudden urge to urinate? Are there certain activities and situations that you avoid for fear of being incontinent?

Worry and Distress

I said at the beginning of this chapter that there are *three* main groups of symptoms associated with bladder problems—frequency, discomfort and incontinence. We have begun to consider what these are and whether they are a problem for you. There still is, however, a huge piece of the picture missing that is rarely talked about—and this can be the key to gaining control over your symptoms. It is how you *feel* about what is happening. You will remember from the "Introduction" how thoughts and feelings about your symptoms can affect how you deal with them as well as their outcome.

We know that having bladder problems can be stressful. In fact, stress can become a major problem in itself. This tension can play a part in prolonging the difficulties, since the bladder is extremely sensitive to stress. Everyone who has been anxious (for example, before taking a driving test or as you are about to give a speech at a business luncheon) can testify to the effect stress has on the bladder.

Are stress and worry playing a major part in your bladder problems? Is the problem on your mind most of the time? Do you feel that it rules your life? Have you enjoyed activities *less*, as a result of bladder problems? Do you routinely avoid certain situations? Do you have difficulty sleeping through the night? Have you told anyone how you feel? I will return to these issues throughout the book.

What Next?

Now that I have introduced the main symptoms of irritable bladder syndrome, think about three important steps before beginning any program to improve your symptoms.

The First Step

I have started you thinking about the kinds of symptoms you have and how they might be affecting you. As I have said, one of the keys to success is understanding your difficulties and making changes. I am going to ask you to keep records of your symptoms, both to understand the possible mechanisms involved and to make changes in what you do. All this requires hard work if you are going to be successful—just reading this book will not in itself change things. However, if reading this book *does* change what you do and how you feel, you are on the road to coping successfully. Remember the old saying, "A journey of a thousand miles begins with the first step."

One of the things that can hold you back is the way you see your problem.

Ways of thinking that will hold you back:

- ◆ Thinking that the problem is your fault
- ◆ Thinking that nothing can be done
- ◆ Thinking that people will judge you harshly

- ◆ Thinking that you can't cope with the embarrassment of going to the doctor

- ◆ Thinking that the problem makes you less of a person

- ◆ Thinking of all the things you can't do

- ◆ Blaming yourself for your bladder problems

Ask yourself:

- ◆ If my best friend told me she had a bladder problem, would I think less of her?

- ◆ What would I advise her to do?

- ◆ Would I feel the same if the problem was, for example, a broken leg?

- ◆ What action would I take for any other physical problem?

- ◆ What can I do?

Ways of thinking that encourage you:

- ◆ Wanting to understand what the problem is

- ◆ Wanting to make changes that will improve the situation

- ◆ Being able to tell someone honestly how you feel about the problem

- ◆ Getting the help you need

- ◆ Doing what you can

- ◆ Telling yourself how well you are doing

The Second Step

The second step is to begin keeping records for yourself. Decide whether or not you have difficulty with frequency, pain, incontinence, or any combination of these, so that you know what to record.

Keep a diary sheet, like the one shown in Figure 1.1 (you can simply photocopy this page), for a week in order to give you a "baseline" to

DIARY SHEET							
	Sun	Mon	Tues	Wed	Thur	Fri	Sat
6 a.m.							
7 a.m.							
8 a.m.							
9 a.m.							
10 a.m.							
11 a.m.							
12 p.m.							
1 p.m.							
2 p.m.							
3 p.m.							
4 p.m.							
5 p.m.							
6 p.m.							
7 p.m.							
8 p.m.							
9 p.m.							
10 p.m.							
11 p.m.							
12 p.m.							
1-5 a.m.							

Figure 1.1 *A weekly diary sheet for monitoring bladder symptoms.*

work from. This will give you time to read through the rest of the book and prepare yourself for any changes you decide to make. I have given you two columns for each day and divided each day into hours. You might wish to make your own version. For example, if you want to record frequency, pain and incontinence, you might want three columns; or if you get up a lot at night, you might want to break that time down in more detail.

To record *frequency* of bladder emptying, simply check the appropriate box. If you wake up at 8 a.m. on Monday morning and go straight to the toilet, put a check in that box. Of course, you may go more than once in that hour, in which case put more than one check in the box. Every time you empty your bladder record it on the sheet.

To record *discomfort*, rate how bad it is on scale from one to ten: one is no discomfort and ten is severe discomfort or pain.

To record *incontinence,* put a cross in the appropriate box for the time when the incontinence occurs and a rating of small (S), medium (M) or large (L) for the amount lost. Small is just a little, making you damp; medium is a moderate amount, say a tablespoonful; and large is a significant amount, or when your bladder has emptied completely.

The Third Step

We all need support and help to help us deal with our problems and to motivate us to make the changes necessary to gain control over them. If you make the decision to change, you also need to find yourself a helper.

Whom you choose will depend on you and your circumstances. You might ask someone in the family or a close friend. If this seems difficult, you might find it easier to talk to someone more detached, such as a doctor or a nurse practitioner. If you have not discussed your difficulties with anyone, it may be a relief to do so. And I am sure you will be surprised how supportive people can be. Of course, you probably won't want too many people to know; confidentiality is also important, so choose someone you trust. As you continue to read the book and decide what applies to you, it will become clearer how your support person can be of great help.

I have said that people often avoid going to the doctor for bladder problems. They may be too embarrassed, or feel that the problem is too trivial, or think that nothing can be done. The bladder is a part of the body like any other, and most doctors will try to put you at ease and will listen to your concerns. There are effective treatments for most bladder problems; the long-term gain of visiting the doctor in terms of the quality of your life should be weighed against your understandable short-term fears.

Make an appointment to see your doctor if:

- ◆ You have never had your bladder difficulties assessed by a doctor.

- ◆ You notice any sudden changes in bladder function.

- ◆ You have any other symptoms, even if they seem unrelated to the bladder.

- ◆ You notice blood in your urine.

- ◆ Urinating is painful.

- ◆ You feel the need to empty your bladder immediately after you have just emptied it.

- ◆ It is difficult to urinate, or the flow is slow or interrupted.

- ◆ You have continuous incontinence.

- ◆ You are very distressed by your bladder problems.

The medical tests, treatments and terminology that you may come across are discussed in Chapter 3.

Summary

I have started to describe the kinds of bladder symptoms that are commonly experienced. As you think about your own situation in light of the information presented thus far, I hope that you will begin to keep clear records of your own particular symptoms. The three main kinds of bladder symptoms were introduced—frequency/ urgency, discomfort and incontinence. Keeping a diary will give you a clear picture of your own symptoms. Making changes can be hard work—so make sure you have the support you need.

CHAPTER TWO

Causes of Bladder Symptoms

We get concerned when we notice changes in how our bodies are working. These changes or "symptoms" can be caused by any number of factors. Understanding your symptoms will lessen your concern and make it clearer how to cope with them. Not all symptoms, particularly those of irritable bladder, are caused by a disease process or medical condition. Remember that the symptoms of irritable bladder problems include a feeling of needing to urinate (urgency), urinating more often than normal (frequency), sometimes feelings of discomfort and, for some people, incontinence. However, several of these same symptoms can occur in other conditions, which I will also discuss.

In this chapter I begin by describing normal bladder functioning. It is then easy to describe how the symptoms of frequency, urgency, discomfort and incontinence can arise. I will describe the groups of symptoms that indicate the particular conditions, and will discuss the current thinking about causes of bladder problems. Tests and treatments are discussed in the next chapter.

Normal Bladder Functioning

At its most basic level, the bladder is a collecting point for urine, which it stores until there is a convenient time and place to urinate. Urine is produced by the kidneys and travels down the ureters into the bladder (see Figure 2.1). The kidneys serve the function of helping the body to regulate the amount of water and salt in the body. If you drink a lot of water, your kidneys will filter off the excess; this process takes about one to two hours. If you drink very little fluid, or are losing water in other ways, such as sweating on a hot day, then less, more-concentrated urine is produced.

As more urine enters the bladder, the bladder wall, which is actually a muscle, relaxes to allow more urine to be stored. Most adult bladders do not need to be emptied more than every two to four hours and can store around 400 to 600 milliliters (14 fluid ounces to 1 pint) of urine. Fill a measuring cup with water to see how much this is (1 fluid pint = 2 cups). Also, try collecting your urine on a couple of

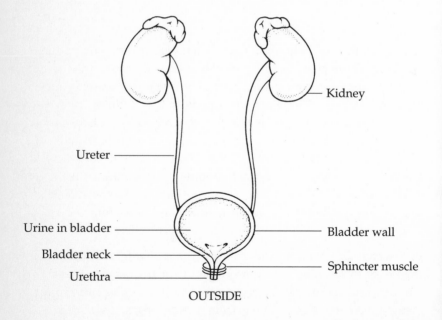

Figure 2.1 *Urine produced in the kidneys travels down the ureters to the bladder.*

occasions in a plastic measuring cup to see how much fluid you typically hold in your bladder. Urine is normally sterile and odorless as it leaves the body, so all you have to do is give the cup a good wash afterward.

As the bladder relaxes on filling, the muscle at the bottom of the bladder contracts to keep the urethra shut so that the urine is contained. It's somewhat like a balloon filled with water that is being pinched at the bottom to keep the water in. It's also similar to your stomach, in that at a certain point you become aware of a feeling of fullness. In the case of the bladder's filling, you then feel the urge to urinate.

The bladder-emptying process is the opposite of the filling one. On filling, the bladder relaxes and the opening contracts; on emptying, the bladder contracts to expel the urine, and the sphincter muscle at the opening relaxes to allow the urine to flow out.

The actual control of this process is rather complicated. What is interesting is that, like some other bodily functions, bladder control is a combination of automatic (reflex) and voluntary (or learned) responses.

Reflex responses are *not* under voluntary control. For example, if the doctor taps your knee in the right place, your leg jerks out of your control; if air is puffed at your eye, you will blink. In babies, bladder emptying is purely reflexive. The bladder fills with urine and at a certain state of fullness the nerves send a message that allows the bladder to contract. It is only later in development that the ability to control this reflex is gained, and that urination can be delayed until convenient. Other bodily functions that are also part automatic reflex and part voluntary are breathing and swallowing. Both are processes that work perfectly naturally, but can also come under conscious control. Have you noticed that once you start paying attention to your breathing it seems to alter it and make it feel unnatural? Could this also apply to your bladder problem? These kinds of bodily processes are often the ones affected by emotional factors, such as worry or stress. For example, worry can lead to fast, shallow breathing and a feeling of tightness in the throat; worry can also lead to the need to urinate. I will discuss these issues in greater depth in Chapter 4.

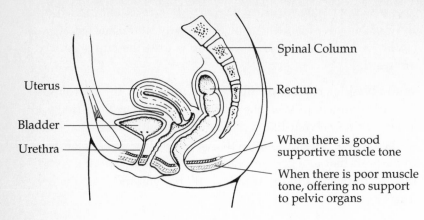

Figure 2.2 *The position of the pelvic floor muscle.*

A few more things about bladder functioning that are relevant to us. They have to do with the importance of the pelvic floor muscles (see Figure 2.2) and the differences between men and women.

The pelvic floor muscles play an important role in bladder functioning. They help the opening of the bladder to stay shut as it fills with urine. The pelvic floor muscles support the pelvic organs—the bladder, the uterus (in women) and the bowel—in a kind of sling. If the muscles are damaged in any way, such as by childbirth or surgery, this can lead to bowel and bladder problems like constipation and incontinence. Similarly, if the muscles are overtensed, perhaps due to habit or in response to pain, then difficulties in urinating can ensue. The next time you empty your bladder try to stop the stream in mid-flow. The muscles you use to do this are the pelvic floor muscles. Did you feel them tighten up? If it was difficult to stop the flow, then it may be that your pelvic floor muscles are rather weak. Do not repeat this "stop" exercise too often because it is important that you always empty your bladder completely.

The role of the pelvic floor muscles is often of particular importance for women with bladder problems, but men, too, have pelvic floor muscles that can be damaged by surgery, such as prostrate surgery. In terms of urinating, women tend to rely to some extent on raising abdominal pressure by bearing down to squeeze the bladder. In men there is more emphasis on the muscle at the neck of the bladder. This means men can more easily "shut off" the flow of urine once it is underway by using this muscle. But conversely, some men have difficulty *starting* bladder emptying, especially when they are anxious.

Now that we know a little about the normal functioning of the bladder, what can go wrong?

Incontinence

There are a number of kinds of incontinence, and the causes can be quite varied.

Stress Incontinence

This has to do with physical rather than emotional stress. Urine is lost on physical exertion, such as coughing, sneezing, laughing, bike riding, jumping or running. What happens is that the muscles that normally keep the bladder opening closed have been unable to do so due to the increased pressure (stress) caused by the physical movement. Try coughing gently and you will be able to feel the strain on the abdomen and pelvic floor. Usually the amount of urine lost due to stress incontinence is small. It is, of course, inconvenient, and people who experience it may avoid certain activities such as sports.

Stress incontinence can be caused by a weakness either of the actual sphincter (the ring of muscle that closes the urethra) or of the pelvic floor muscles (which support the bladder). Problems can be triggered by trauma to the area; the most typical examples are childbirth and surgery.

If you lose urine immediately on exertion, you probably have stress incontinence. Build up the courage to speak to your doctor about it if you have not already done so (your doctor will not be shocked or ashamed of you, I assure you!). The most common treatment for stress incontinence is pelvic floor exercises, which are often very effective (see Chapter 7). Surgery may be recommended for severe cases, but only when more conservative treatments have failed.

Overflow Incontinence

This is the opposite of stress incontinence. Rather than urine escaping too easily from the bladder, the bladder-emptying mechanism is obstructed in some way. Once the bladder is full, the high pressure forces the urine out in a steady dribble.

Enlargement of the prostate gland in men can obstruct bladder emptying. The other possibility is that there is an abnormal hole somewhere that allows urine to escape. Obviously, you need medical attention for these symptoms, if you have them, and you should see your doctor.

Irritable Bladder Problems

The various problems described below are those I generally term "irritable bladder," which are different from those where there is a clear cause, such as infection. This is because they involve the symptoms of frequency and urgency described earlier, and are often made worse by stress.

Urge Incontinence

Urge incontinence has more to do with the behavior of the bladder muscle itself than either stress or overflow incontinence. This kind of incontinence always involves a strong sensation of the urge to empty the bladder, accompanied by a loss of urine.

One cause of urge incontinence is that the bladder muscle contracts as it would to empty the bladder, despite the person's attempts to inhibit that action. This is more correctly called "motor urge incontinence." The amount of urine lost is usually large—often the entire contents of the bladder. This kind of "bladder instability," as it is also known, can only be properly assessed by appropriate tests. Sometimes the bladder contractions can be triggered by physical events, such as coughing or violent sneezing, but there is a delay between the event and the incontinence. This kind of incontinence is also associated with bedwetting (enuresis), which is when the bladder-voiding reflex occurs during sleep.

Bladder instability can also be caused by obstructions such as an enlarged prostate gland or bladder stones.

If you have these kinds of symptoms, make an appointment with your physician to discuss them before embarking on a self-help program. There is often no obvious physical reason for the bladder's contracting in this way. The bladder is affected by many different factors, not all of them physical (see Chapter 4).

Sometimes there can be incontinence and a sense of urgency without there being actual bladder contractions; this is more correctly termed "sensory urge incontinence." Usually the amount of urine lost is little.

Motor and sensory urge incontinence, including bedwetting, tend to respond well to bladder-training procedures, which are described in Chapter 7.

Urgency and Frequency

These are obviously associated with the urge incontinence problems described above. However, they also often exist on their own, without incontinence. This syndrome has many names and causes, but the essential element is a sensitive bladder that is often uncomfortable because of the feeling of urgency. This syndrome compels the sufferer to visit the bathroom frequently and to lead a life that is ruled by his or her bladder problems.

Ironically, sufferers are rarely incontinent, but often live in fear of this possibility and restrict their lifestyles accordingly. If you follow the procedures described in this book, you will have an excellent chance of overcoming your difficulties, over time.

There can be underlying factors associated with chronic urgency and frequency, such as a low-grade infection of some kind; this possibility should be excluded by having the correct medical tests and treatment before doing anything else.

Pain and Discomfort

When urgency and frequency, and possibly incontinence, are associated with pain—particularly if there is pain while urinating—you probably have an infection. You should, of course, seek out appropriate treatment.

Most people have heard of cystitis, a term often used to describe bladder infections. Usually such infections are simply caused by bacteria from the bowel entering the bladder, but occasionally they may be caused by other problems, such as bladder stones.

Cystitis is far more common in women than men, with 10 percent of women suffering from it each year. This is because the urethra in women is close to the anus and the bacteria only have a short distance to travel up the urethra to the bladder. Cystitis can also be caused by other organisms, however. Infections are usually fairly short-lived and can sometimes be cured by drinking copious amounts of water to flush out the bacteria. You should always consult your doctor if the symptoms last more than a day, if you have blood in your urine or if there are other symptoms such as fever.

Evidence suggests that some women are prone to suffering recurrent bouts of cystitis. This can be very stressful and debilitating. Your doctor should be able to help you find the most appropriate treatment, and should be willing to approve your using a number of self-help procedures that are very effective. The key points to remember are: drink plenty of bland fluid (especially water); empty your bladder every two hours; keep the vaginal area clean; and empty the bladder before and after sex. Also, follow the general advice given in Chapters 5 to 10 of this book. There are some excellent self-help books on the topic of recurrent cystitis—see the "Further Reading" section at the end of the book.

If you suffer from urgency, frequency and pain all the time, it is likely that you have been told you have interstitial cystitis. This is an inflammation of the lining of the bladder, similar to a stomach ulcer.

Some authorities disagree about the cause of this syndrome, and it is likely that there are a number of different ones. Certain researchers argue that the cause has to do with an infection, while others believe the syndrome is caused by a disorder of the immune system. Mild symptoms can be helped by the procedures described in Chapters 5 to 10; those who are suffering severe symptoms are sometimes offered surgery.

Often, bladder problems are associated not with the acute, sharp pain of an infection, but rather with chronic aches and discomfort that comes and goes. Incontinence and irritable bladder are associated with a range of other symptoms. Sufferers often also have irritable bowel problems, recurrent headaches and backaches, as well as discomfort in the lower abdomen.

If physical causes for these symptoms have been eliminated by the proper tests, it is likely that they are stress related. Many of my patients are initially mystified at how stress can cause pain. But remember, one of the first things that happens when you feel stressed is that you tense up. People tend to get tense in different ways; some suffer from headaches because their neck muscles are tensed up. If you are tense about your bladder (the expression "uptight" says it all), it makes sense that you will tense up around the pelvic area, which can over time lead to aches and pains. If you doubt that muscle tension can cause pain, think of the agony of a leg cramp, which is just acute muscle tension! If you think this may apply to you, read Chapters 5 to 10 carefully.

Summary

I have covered some basic information about how the bladder works and what can go wrong. I hope that this has helped you make more sense of the symptoms that you have been suffering. In the next chapter, I will describe the kinds of medical tests that are currently available, as well as common treatments.

CHAPTER THREE

Medical Tests, Treatments and Terms

I mentioned earlier that you should make an appointment to see your physician, if you have not already done so. I know that many people are reluctant to visit the doctor, and tend to put off making the call. When you ask people—particularly incontinence sufferers—why this is, they give a number of reasons. They are often unclear whether or not bladder difficulties represent a legitimate medical concern; they feel that their problems are an almost inevitable price to pay for getting older, having babies, exercising vigorously or whatever. They may also feel a great deal of embarrassment at the thought of discussing these problems and are unsure of the reception they will receive. It is as if people hide such difficulties as a way of coping; they think if they don't talk about the symptoms, they're not really a problem. Often, close friends and family are unaware of the extent of someone's difficulties, compounding one's feelings of isolation and being different.

Are you putting off getting the appropriate help and support for these reasons? The situation is unlikely to improve if you ignore it. In fact, quite the opposite can be true. Why put up with troublesome symptoms if effective help is readily available? I will try to give you a good idea of the kinds of things to expect when you visit your doctor—what he or she will ask you, the kinds of examinations and tests you may have to undertake and the treatments he or she might suggest. I will also describe the kinds of investigations you might experience if you are referred to a urologist. At the back of the book is a glossary of some of the medical terms you might come across.

Going to See Your Doctor

The first step is to make an appointment. Consider ways to make this as easy on yourself as possible. Allow adequate time, take a friend along to wait with you if you find this helpful, or take a good book or magazine to distract you and calm your nerves as you wait to talk to your doctor.

If you have been putting off going to the doctor because he is a male and you would prefer to see a woman (or perhaps the opposite if you are a man), you have a number of options. Doctors see a large number of people with bladder problems, so, with luck, male and female doctors should be equally sympathetic. If you belong to a group practice or a health maintenance organization (HMO), then ask to see the person (or someone of the gender) you would feel most at ease with. There is no need to tell the receptionist why you are making this request; all medical conversations are confidential. Remember, you are probably a hundred-fold more uncomfortable about this consultation than your doctor; it is routine for them. If you are particularly anxious, it might be worth mentioning this to the doctor so that he or she can do his or her best to put you at ease.

Once you are with the doctor, mention any specific fears you might have, such as anxieties about needles or blood. If these are a problem for you, you may need help to tackle them. Phobias like these can be easily conquered, given the correct help and support. Ask your doctor to recommend someone who can help you. In my work I have seen many people overcome these kinds of fears in a matter of weeks, and they feel much more confident because of this.

Your doctor will find it very helpful if you have been keeping a diary of your symptoms. The pattern of your symptoms will help them to decide on the next steps to take. Take your completed copy of the diary on page 7 with you when you go.

You will probably be asked to provide a urine specimen. If you would rather take this with you than have to produce one at the office, then either drop into the office before the appointment to pick up a specimen bottle or use any clean, watertight container (slip it into a lock-tight plastic bag to carry it to the doctor's office). You only need to collect a few ounces, but make sure the sample is a "mid-stream" one. This means you need to start urinating, stop the flow if you can and then collect your sample in the middle of the flow. As you might imagine, this can be a bit tricky!

The specimen is needed to check whether or not there is any infection in the bladder. The results of the test will take a few days to come back. The doctor may also test whether there is sugar in the urine (to check for diabetes) or blood in the urine. They can usually do these latter two tests at the office.

Write down the details of all medications that you take, especially if you are not seeing your usual doctor.

If you have kept a diary and have been thinking about your symptoms, you will be able to easily answer questions about frequency/ urgency, discomfort and incontinence. Your doctor may also ask questions about other aspects of your health and is likely to examine you. You may have your blood pressure taken or the doctor may want to do a blood test to check the levels of certain hormones and other substances in your system. In terms of physical examinations, the doctor will probably want to feel your abdomen to check for any abnormalities. They will also want to do a rectal and (if you're a woman) vaginal examination to check for abnormalities, constipation or infection. This is probably the most anxiety-provoking part of the procedure, but it is essential if the doctor is to arrive at the right conclusions and to eliminate the possibility of there being any structural problems. Try to relax if you feel uptight at this stage. Remember that you are free to ask the doctor to explain fully what he or she is doing, to stop at any time (particularly if you feel any discomfort) and to take someone in with you if you want to.

Treatment

The doctor may ask to see you again to discuss the results of the tests, may refer you to a specialist or may recommend some form of treatment. The doctor may refer you to a physiotherapist for pelvic floor exercises if they think that pelvic floor weakness is contributing to your difficulties. (See Chapter 7.)

Another possibility is that you will be prescribed some medication, in the form of tablets. If you have urge incontinence, you may be prescribed oxybutynin. The effect of this is to reduce uncontrolled bladder contractions. A similar drug is imipramine, which needs to be taken for about a week if you are to notice a therapeutic effect.

Drugs act on the whole body and often cause some side effects. For treatment to be effective, the drugs have to be taken in such potent dosages that you are almost certain to notice other effects. These can include a dry mouth, blurred vision, increased heart rate and flushing. You may also feel drowsy, dizzy or nauseated or may get constipated. People are affected differently by side effects, which tend to improve over time. Some people find the treatment difficult to tolerate; if this applies to you, keep a note of any symptoms and report back to your physician. If you develop a difficulty in passing urine, contact your doctor immediately.

Although drugs used for bladder control problems are not addictive, they *do* act on your nervous system. Medications may help symptoms, and for some people they sort the problem out, but in the long run you need to cope without them. If you plan to embark on a self-help program, ask your doctor if you can initially go without drugs, to allow your bladder to be trained under normal circumstances; you will have a better chance of long-term success.

Sometimes muscle relaxants or tranquilizers are prescribed for problems such as sensory urgency. Again, this may help in the short term, but these drugs are addictive and are not for long-term use. Why not try the program in this book or ask what advice the doctor can give other than drug therapy? Always make sure you understand (and write down if you are likely to forget) the name of the drug being prescribed, its mode of action—for example, is it a tranquilizer?—and its likely side effects.

Other forms of medication may include an antibiotic or antifungal agent if you have an infection, or hormone replacement therapy if your doctor thinks this may help your symptoms. Remember that finding the right treatment is a collaborative venture. You need to give the doctor accurate information and feedback about whether or not the treatment prescribed is working. You should be able to discuss the alternatives to medication; it may be that drug therapy is not appropriate. Your doctor may give you some general advice about bladder training, fluid intake and diet, and can help you combine these approaches with medication.

Going to the Hospital

If you are referred to a urologist—a physician who specializes in the urinary or urogenital tract—you may undergo additional tests. Again, take along your diary and a note of any medication, and be prepared to provide a urine specimen—don't empty your bladder before you see the doctor!

The following description will give you a general idea of what will happen. Each specialist, however, will vary one from the other. You should be given a full explanation of any procedures by the staff; if in doubt, ask. Some urologists will have a portable ultrasound machine (like the ones used for showing mothers-to-be a scan of their unborn babies), which will allow the doctor to see the bladder and such problems as bladder stones.

If blood was found in your urine, then you may have to have a cystoscopy. This is a fairly simple outpatient procedure (done under local anesthesia) where a tiny camera within a fine tube is inserted into the bladder so that the doctor can see if there is any abnormality, such as inflammation or a growth.

Urodynamic studies (or cystometry) involve a series of tests to assess the behavior of the bladder on filling and emptying. These are usually recommended when there is a mixture of symptoms, an operation is being considered or previous treatment has not been effective. You are usually asked to come with a full bladder and to urinate (in private) into a special commode that records the amount of urine you pass and the rate at which it flows. The next stage is completed while you are lying down. A small tube (catheter) is passed into the bladder; this will be used to fill the bladder. Another fine tube will also be inserted that measures pressure, and another one is inserted into the rectum to measure abdominal pressure. Although you may feel some discomfort while the catheters are being put into place, it is usually mild and passes quickly. The bladder is then slowly filled with fluid and you will be asked to indicate when you first get the desire to empty your bladder, and then again when you feel that you really must go. The filling tube is then removed and you will be asked to stand and move or cough. Finally, you will be asked to empty your bladder so that volume and flow can again be recorded. After the pressure recorders are removed, the procedure is complete.

I know this test doesn't sound pleasant, but it *does* allow a proper assessment to be made of how well the bladder is functioning; be assured that the staff will explain each part of the procedure. Again, if you are feeling tense, try to practice a relaxation technique (or listen to a favorite meditation tape) before the appointment. You will usually know beforehand that you will have a certain procedure and will be given all the information you need to prepare yourself for it.

Treatment

The urologist may recommend the same kind of drug treatment your general practitioner might offer, or physiotherapy (if there is weakness of the pelvic floor muscles), or an intensive course of bladder retraining, or perhaps surgery in extreme cases. Bladder retraining may take place either on an out- or in-patient basis and is fundamentally an intensive course to re-educate the bladder (the basics of bladder retraining are considered in Chapter 7). Surgery may involve repairing the pelvic floor, correcting a prolapse of any of the pelvic organs or repairing a weakness in the bladder neck. Sometimes there is an obstruction in the bladder or urethra that needs to be removed, or, in males, an enlarged prostate gland may be hindering urination and it needs to be removed. Also, if less invasive treatments for an unstable bladder have failed, then surgery is sometimes recommended. This might involve interrupting the nerve supply to the bladder wall or inserting a piece of bowel material into the bladder wall to make it larger. All surgery has potential drawbacks, and you should be sure you understand what is being recommended, what the alternatives and risks are and why the surgery (rather than something else) is considered to be the next step. It is, of course, only a minority of people who will end up having any kind of surgery.

Two final procedures that are now more rarely used for bladder problems and are sometimes recommended for sensory urgency or interstitial cystitis are the stretching of the urethra (by inserting various-sized tubes into it) or stretching of the bladder (by overfilling it with fluid for a longish period). There are risks associated with such procedures, and it is not clear whether people truly benefit from them in the long run. Again, make sure you know the pros and cons of *any* procedure that is recommended.

What Next?

If you have consulted your doctor and have a good idea about your particular difficulties, then you likely will have a better idea of how to overcome them. You may have been given certain treatments and advice and can enhance these by following the appropriate sections of the program of bladder training, pelvic floor exercises and general lifestyle changes that I will go on to describe.

CHAPTER FOUR

Physical and Emotional Factors and the Bladder

The bladder is a sensitive beast! Its functioning can be influenced by a whole range of factors. Fortunately, most of these factors are directly under your control, or can be improved by taking the appropriate action. As with most things in life, it is usually the case that there is no single, simple "cause" of bladder difficulties that can be fixed immediately by a doctor. Usually such difficulties worsen over time, perhaps for a number of reasons, and require a "multifaceted" approach. I hope to describe as many things that can affect bladder functioning as possible, and to illustrate how these factors come to interact so that symptoms are managed over time.

Diet

The idea that your diet can influence your bladder may seem slightly odd. It is the *effects* of your diet that are important. For example, chronic constipation can result from your diet and may cause problems. Remember that the rectum and the bladder are close together and are both supported by the pelvic floor muscles. Straining to have a bowel movement stretches and weakens these muscles. If constipation is a constant problem for you, then it may be advisable to seek medical help. If it is only occasionally a problem, then it is a good idea to pay special attention to your diet. The most common causes of constipation are a lack of fiber in the diet, not enough exercise, ignoring the need to empty the bowel, and certain drugs. Drinking too little fluid may also be a factor.

Being overweight is another adverse influence of your diet; the bladder is supported by the pelvic floor, which can be overworked if you are obese.

Some say that certain kinds of foods, such as very spicy ones, can influence the bladder. It is probably advisable to avoid salty foods, because too much salt can be dehydrating. In general, try to follow the advice given in Chapter 8.

Drinks

It's probably a little easier to see the connection between what you drink and your bladder—the link is more direct. Most of us don't drink enough fluid and don't drink the right things, but rectifying this situation is important if you have a bladder problem.

At all costs, resist the temptation to reduce your intake of fluids as a way of coping with frequency and urgency. This is not good for your health in general and merely trains your bladder to cope with less and less fluid over time; that is, you are making it *more* sensitive, not less. The recommended daily intake of fluid is about 8 to 10 glasses of water a day, or around 3 pints. This seems like a lot, but it is easiest if you increase your intake slowly. Many of the people I have seen who have been able to manage this had once reduced their intake to small sips, or about *one* glass a day—dangerously insufficient.

The other major factor is *what* you drink. The most important thing to avoid is caffeine (in coffee, some teas, and many soft drinks, including "diet" brands). This is a stimulant and has a very marked effect on bladder sensitivity! Other drinks to avoid in excess include alcohol (it is dehydrating), concentrated fruit juices and carbonated canned or bottled drinks, which are acidic.

(See Chapter 6 for more detailed information and advice on fluid intake.)

Health

Other general health factors that may influence the bladder include coughing, lifting, medication and infections. Chronic coughing can be a problem, because each time you cough you increase both your abdominal pressure and the strain on the pelvic floor, which in the long term can affect the bladder. Repeated heavy lifting can also put a strain on the pelvic floor. Try to avoid heavy lifting or consciously tighten the pelvic muscles as you lift.

Certain kinds of drugs for other medical problems, such as diuretics (commonly known as "water tablets") for high blood pressure, can alter bladder functioning. Bladder infections such as cystitis—particularly, recurrent attacks—can increase the sensitivity of the bladder in general. Just getting older can have an influence on the bladder and lead to other problems, such as having to get up several times at night to urinate.

A number of bladder problems can be overcome, or at least greatly relieved, by following the self-help advice given in this book, particularly the pelvic floor exercises, which can improve things at any age. Regaining pelvic and abdominal muscle tone by means of appropriate exercises is a major step in the right direction.

Differences Between Women and Men

For women, there are certain events and influences in life that are important and may act as the starting point for bladder trouble. Pregnancy, childbirth or a hysterectomy all affect the bladder, even if only for the short term. Obviously they affect the abdomen and pelvic floor where the bladder is located and supported. Hormonal changes may also be important, and, indeed, many women find that their bladder symptoms vary with their menstrual cycle. Also, some women report symptoms when menopause begins. The important thing to remember is that you should keep a diary of symptoms, consult your doctor where appropriate and follow the general advice in this book.

Although on the whole men have fewer bladder problems, it is not unusual for men too to suffer incontinence and irritable bladder symptoms. Apart from the factors described immediately above, which relate to women, the other causes of bladder problems mentioned so far, such as obesity and constipation, apply equally to men and women. The one particular physical factor that applies solely to men is the prostate gland. This gland is at the base of the bladder and the urethra passes through it. If the prostate gland becomes enlarged, which often happens with age, the urethra becomes restricted and even blocked. The symptoms associated with this happening are:

- Frequency
- Discomfort urinating
- Difficulty starting to urinate, and a slow stream
- Dribbling incontinence
- Having to get up at night to urinate.

Your doctor will arrange for appropriate tests if it is thought that this is a problem for you, and you may be advised to have a prostatectomy. This can be done in various ways and you may only need a local anesthetic for the surgery. Ask about any questions or concerns you have. Men commonly experience some bladder symptoms following the operation. Pelvic floor exercises may be helpful in improving bladder control; these are described in Chapter 7.

One other problem can be a difficulty for men, although women may also suffer from it. This is difficulty in starting to urinate, or "retention" of urine. This may only occur in particular circumstances. For example, quite a large proportion of men find it difficult to urinate alongside others in a public restroom. Hardly surprising, really!

This phenomenon is sometimes called "bashful bladder." It may be an occasional or mild problem, causing little disruption to everyday life; or it can develop over time until it becomes very restricting. I have talked to someone whose difficulties had generalized to include any public restrooms, such that train trips and an evening spent drinking with friends at a bar were major sources of anxiety. Again, my advice is *not* to restrict your fluids as a way of coping with this. Instead, learn a relaxation technique and talk yourself through it when you are having difficulty urinating, taking the pressure off yourself to perform. If you cannot go after a minute or so, give up and try later. Sometimes trying *not* to go will actually help!

Occasionally difficulties urinating can be brought on by a severe shock or trauma—for example, the death of a loved one or experiencing an accident. This leads us into a discussion of psychological factors that can affect the bladder.

Psychological Factors

The bladder often reflects the way we are feeling. One of the symptoms of anxiety and stress is an increased feeling of urgency, hence the frequent visits to the restroom before a big event such as a wedding or a college reunion dinner. No one really understands the exact mechanism behind this, but it is similar to the experience of "butterflies" in the stomach. Our bodies are very much affected by our psychological state. Stress and anxiety are individual things—no two people experience the same event in the same way. Sometimes bladder problems date back to a time of "acute" stress, such as a bereavement, or to a more prolonged strain such as ongoing marital, financial or work worries. Is this the case for you?

Whatever the initial triggers of bladder problems may be, they can then be maintained by other factors. Consider the following. A person is under a lot of stress at work and home, and the increased levels of anxiety lead to increased feelings of urgency and hence frequent urinating. Not making the link between the anxiety and these symptoms, the person begins to wonder about their cause. The nature of this wondering depends on their personal experiences. The woman whose mother had distressing problems of incontinence and confusion before she died may fear a loss of control. The man who has an uncle with prostate trouble may fear physical illness. The sense that these people make of their difficulties then influences their actions. The woman might reduce her intake of fluids and increase the number of times she goes to the bathroom, to (in her mind) reduce the risk of an "accident." She is then likely to become very aware of any sensations of fullness in her bladder. Her anxiety, therefore, would not be allayed and her strategies would actually increase her bladder sensitivity over time, leading to more worry about symptoms and more attempts to control them. Can you see the vicious circle that develops? The man might visit the doctor and be referred for tests. He then might think that the doctor must think there is something wrong. The tests may come back negative, although he still has the symptoms. He might then think that he may have something "worse" and ask for more tests. He might monitor his symptoms, worry about their significance and find that the anxiety leads to more symptoms, confirming in his mind the presence of a serious problem. Another vicious circle is created. Regardless of how the original stress progresses, the bladder symptoms are now under the influence of each person's thoughts and behavior.

Anxiety about other things, or the symptoms themselves, can make bladder problems worse (see Figure 4.1). The signs of stress and anxiety are more fully explained in Chapter 9, but it is worth saying here that paying attention to the symptoms can indeed make them worse. When I give talks on this topic, people often tell me afterward that the more I spoke about frequency, urgency and incontinence, the more they felt the need to go to the bathroom. In fact, reading this book may make you pay more attention to your bladder and hence experience more sensation. You can test out this idea yourself. Spend two minutes or so thinking about bladder sensations and concentrating on your bladder, and then, on a scale of one to ten, rate how much

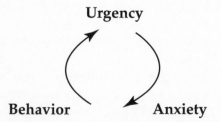

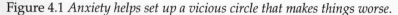

Figure 4.1 *Anxiety helps set up a vicious circle that makes things worse.*

of an urge to go to the bathroom you felt while doing this. Then go off and read a column in the newspaper or a page in a book as if someone were going to ask you questions about it afterward. Rate the urgency you felt again at the end of this time, without thinking about it too long. I hope you see the difference. Distraction techniques are described in Chapter 10; they help you focus attention away from your bladder so that the sensations are easier to cope with.

The bladder is "suggestible"—if you think about having to go to the bathroom, you will want to go (just as you likely will yawn if you see someone else do so, even on television). And the bladder is sensitive to anxiety and worry, and to too much attention. It is also a creature of habit. If you always go to the toilet at a certain time, the bladder becomes trained and you may feel urgency in this situation, whether the bladder is full or not. Sometimes these patterns are established in early childhood. My parents—and they were not alone—were in the habit of putting me on the toilet before we went out and running water to encourage me to urinate. To this day, for a lot of people, the sound of running water triggers the need to urinate! (I, for one, am a little wary of visiting scenic waterfalls.) This is a process of learning links between events, and it goes on throughout our lives. It is possible to unlearn these links by not succumbing to the urge. Each time you do this it becomes easier—believe me.

Summary

Various factors influence bladder functioning. I hope you can identify those that apply to you, so that you can go on to make the kinds of changes that will reduce irritable bladder symptoms and give you back control over your life.

CHAPTER FIVE

Pain and Discomfort

Issues of pain and discomfort are rather complex. There are a number of possible reasons for experiencing such difficulties with bladder problems, some of which I have already touched on. The other essential consideration is that the experience of pain and discomfort is never simply related to physical factors. I will explain and illustrate this point.

Have you ever injured yourself, even if it's only slightly, and not actually noticed until some time after the event? To take an example from my own experience, I remember going rock climbing (for the first and last time!) with some friends and being so focused on getting to the top of the cliff that I did not notice I had scraped some skin off the back of my hand until a few minutes after achieving my goal. Driven by adrenaline and excitement, I did not feel the pain at all during the climb. Under other circumstances, if I'd grazed my hand I would have felt the pain immediately. There are even more dramatic examples of this phenomenon, such as athletes who break bones during the course of an important event and do not feel pain until after the game is over. This phenomenon occurs because the feeling of pain is influenced *both* by the messages from the nerves in the affected part of the body being sent up to the brain *and* by the messages from the brain being sent back down to the site of the injury. The messages being sent *down* are related to your emotional and psychological state.

The implication of this is that the same injury can feel different at different times. There is no simple one-to-one relationship between injury and the feeling of pain. Of course, you expect grazes and broken bones to hurt in the short term, and, depending on the seriousness of the injury, this will be more or less distressing. You also expect them to get better over time. Some pain and discomfort, however, does *not* seem to get better over time, and this can be described as chronic pain.

Chronic pain, such as can occasionally apply to bladder problems, is under the influence of even more factors than the acute pain we have been looking at so far. And it is even more complicated. When pain is chronic, it inevitably has a psychological impact. That is, you think, feel and act in a certain way about the pain. The nature of the reaction to chronic pain can influence how you cope; and it can influence the quality of your life. It can also influence those around you, who will in turn react. This, too, can influence the course of the problem, and on and on around an infinite loop. The leap I have just made from a physical pain to a feeling that is influenced by those around you may seem unlikely, but I assure you that this is a common scenario. Here is a typical example of what I mean.

> David had been having bladder trouble for some time. He had sensations of urgency, with difficulty urinating. It was eventually decided that he needed prostate surgery.
>
> David was at a low ebb. His work was physically demanding, stressful and not well paid; it wasn't even secure. This had also led to some strains in his relationship with his wife and children.
>
> After the surgery he was in pain. This made him feel even more depressed, and the thought of going back to work filled him with dread. His wife and kids were very supportive and caring. She made sure he took his painkillers, looked after all his needs and cooked his favorite dishes. His kids made him

cards and presents. If the pain was bad, he would ask for painkillers and go to bed. His wife was particularly attentive and caring at these times. He still felt tense about going back to work, but after a couple of weeks felt he should go back.

While at work on that first day, he did not feel particularly well and experienced an excruciating cramping pain in his lower abdomen. He was sent home. His wife was very concerned, and his doctor gave him a sick note for another week. Over time it became more and more difficult for David to return to work. You can see how a pattern developed that David and his wife found difficult to stop.

Fortunately, David eventually acknowledged his fears about his health and work to his wife, and later to his supervisor and doctor. They worked out a way for him to gradually return to work and to receive all the medical reassurance he needed, while his wife encouraged his positive efforts at slowly getting back to a more balanced lifestyle.

As you can see from this example, chronic pain can be affected by psychological factors and general life circumstances. This is supported by the fact that chronic pain and discomfort can vary in intensity over time. It is important to identify the factors that cause these changes. Some may be already clear to you. For example, many of the people I see can make a definite link between feeling stressed and the discomfort worsening. To get a clear idea of the factors influencing discomfort over time, it is essential to keep a diary. This allows you to pay direct attention to your level of discomfort as it relates to such things as your level of activity, feelings of stress or whatever. You will recall the description of how to keep a diary given in Chapter 1. There you rated your discomfort on a scale of one to ten, initially every hour. Now you can use this diary to take note of what is happening at that time, or include an additional rating of, for example, stress or anxiety if it is relevant to you.

The three main psychological factors of chronic pain are:

- Depression
- Tension
- Attention

Depression

It has been found that those who suffer chronic pain and discomfort are often depressed. Naturally, there has been a chicken-and-egg-type debate about which comes first. Overall, the conclusion seems to be that the two interact together. It is important to recognize if you are depressed, since depression brings on pain sensations and will have an enormous influence on how you are able to tackle your health problems and conduct your daily living. But, be reassured, depression is easily conquered when you are given the appropriate support. What exactly *is* depression?

Do you frequently:

- Feel downhearted and sad?
- Feel at your worst in the morning?
- Have crying spells?
- Have trouble getting to sleep?
- Wake up too early?
- Have no appetite?
- Notice you are losing weight?
- Feel tired or irritable?
- Find it hard to do things?
- Feel hopeless?
- Find it difficult to enjoy anything?

If a few of these symptoms apply to you and you have felt like this for some time, it is important that you visit your doctor to talk about how you have been feeling. The sooner you tackle depression, the better off you will be. Over time it is possible to feel more and more hopeless, and helpless, as a result of the downward spiral that develops; you feel tired and low and do less, which leads to feeling more negative, and so on. Your doctor may suggest that you talk to a therapist or psychologist or may prescribe an antidepressant medication.

Depression is a very common problem, particularly in those with chronic health problems (around 30 to 40 percent of people) and is an understandable reaction to such difficulties. You are not alone, and the problem *can* be solved. Try to determine whether the depression has to do with your bladder problems and came about after these difficulties arose, or whether you were already depressed.

If you feel your life is limited by your symptoms:

> ◆ Take a positive approach to overcoming them.

> ◆ Remind yourself of your achievements and the things you can do.

> ◆ Ask yourself if you are really limited by your symptoms or by your own fears.

> ◆ Remember that having bladder problems in no way affects your worth as a person, unless you let it.

> ◆ Don't dwell on things you can't do or on how things have changed; make positive plans, and take one step at a time.

Other factors in people's lives can add to feelings of depression or a lack of self-worth, such as problems in a significant relationship or stress at work. It could be that ongoing tension of this kind is compounding your bladder symptoms and feelings of depression. (See Chapter 9.)

Some people have experienced very traumatic events, either in childhood or during their adult lives, such as bereavement, a family break-up, a serious accident or illness, or mistreatment at the hands of others. Often they have not had the opportunity to come to terms with what has happened, and they end up feeling stressed and depressed. If you think that this applies to you, it is important that you try to find appropriate help. Doctors and spiritual counselors (such as clergy, priests or rabbis) are aware of the counseling services available to you locally.

Sometimes it is difficult to accept that physical distress is linked to emotional factors, particularly if the memories are very painful. As a psychologist working with people who have chronic health problems, I encounter this every day and am often struck by the fact that people have never told those close to them about the experiences that have had a tremendous impact on their lives and on their feelings. To come to terms with some experiences, it is essential to work with someone else, someone who is experienced and professional, someone you trust.

We have seen that it is possible to feel depressed about adjusting to the limitations your symptoms have brought about. Depression will affect your bladder problems in two ways: making any discomfort feel worse, and making it difficult to cope practically and emotionally. If in your heart of hearts you believe that your bladder problems have ruined your life, or that they affect your worth as a person, you will feel depressed no matter how hard you try to battle them. Admit to yourself if this is how you really feel—and then challenge these ideas by collecting evidence against them.

Another meaning that people give to their symptoms is that they are harmful. This naturally leads to feelings of tension and anxiety. Tension is the second factor that can "turn on" pain and discomfort.

Tension

In addition to depression, you may be feeling tense or stressed. Again, this can be a result of your symptoms ("I wonder if there is something seriously wrong with me..."; "What if I can't find a restroom soon?") or because of other aspects of your life ("It will be a catastrophe if I get fired!"). No matter how the tension and stress have arisen, they make your symptoms and any discomfort worse. Stress is a physical reaction. (See Chapters 9 and 10.)

If you have worries about your symptoms, you probably need some reassurance from your doctor. If you have worries about your bladder's letting you down, follow the self-help advice given in this book. You may also ask yourself "What is the worst thing that could happen?" People often react emotionally because they are thinking how terrible something is: "It would be terrible to be incontinent while I am out shopping." This leads to feeling stressed while you are out, and makes you worried about the state of your bladder, which will in turn lead to more bladder sensations and more worry, and so on (see Figure 5.1).

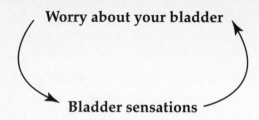

Figure 5.1 *The vicious circle of tension and bladder problems.*

Ask yourself:

- ◆ How likely is the thing I fear?
- ◆ Has it happened before?
- ◆ If it did happen, what would be so terrible?
- ◆ What is it that I really fear?

Often what people really fear is not the event itself, but what the event might mean for them. For example, a sociable person who feels good about himself when his relationships with others are going well and who likes to be seen as a confident, coping person may fear that people will reject him because of his problems. But just think: would your friends actually abandon you under these circumstances? How would *you* react if this happened to someone else? Is this situation truly terrible, or just not very nice? Try to be honest with yourself about what it is that you really fear; then ask yourself is it really likely to happen and would it really be a total catastrophe.

Just as you can get into a downward spiral with depression, you can get into an upward spiral with tension and discomfort. You feel tense because you are in pain, which makes the pain worse, which makes the tension worse, and so on, around and around the vicious circle. The more you worry about the symptoms the worse they get, in part because by worrying about them you are paying attention to them. Attention is the third factor that can "turn on" pain.

Attention

We are only able to pay attention to a fraction of the information that is available to us for consideration at any one time. Also, whatever you are actively attending to will seem in some ways "amplified." For example, if you are sitting watching your favorite TV program, you are *not* thinking about your Aunt Judy, what the weather is like or how much you enjoy eating Thai food. You are focused on the plot and the sounds and the imagery of the TV program, which in turn makes you feel happy, sad or whatever. If Aunt Judy then telephones you to wish you good luck with your daughter's wedding on Saturday, you may start thinking about something else altogether and the TV program then becomes a faint noise in the background.

The same is true about attention and pain. If you are *focusing* on discomfort, it will be all that is in your mind, because it is in the spotlight. If you are distracted by something else, the pain will not be receiving your complete attention, and, for the time being, it will not appear to be as bad. (Techniques for using this distraction to your advantage are described in Chapter 10.)

Summary

If you are suffering pain and discomfort and you have assurance from your doctor that all medical angles have been explored, then you are faced with the prospect of learning to cope with your problems. First, as always, know your enemy. Keep a diary so that you can see what makes the problems better and worse, and then use this knowledge. Is your discomfort influenced by your emotional state? Are you depressed or stressed? What do you need to do to reduce these feelings? Do you focus your attention on the discomfort more than is necessary? Use distraction techniques to change this.

CHAPTER SIX

You Are What You Drink!

Now that you have information about your problem, we will put forth strategies for tackling them. We touched earlier on the importance of drinking enough liquid. You will now find out how to make the necessary changes in your drinking habits. But remember, changing habits, especially if they are ones that are ingrained, should be a slow process. Something that I cannot emphasize enough is that changes made in a steady, progressive way over a period of time are more likely to be permanent than those you try to make overnight. It is a bit like the hare and the tortoise. It is enough that you are moving in the right direction—do not worry if your progress is slow or even if you occasionally take a few steps backward.

Why Drink More Liquid?

There are two main reasons for this. The first concerns your general health. There is more water in our bodies than any other substance. All the major bodily functions work best if the body is well hydrated—

that is to say, when there is enough water. Dehydration can lead to headaches, constipation and other health problems.

The second reason for drinking plenty is more specific and concerns your bladder. The bladder also works best when you are drinking the right amount of fluid. If you drink too little, then the bladder gets used to holding smaller and smaller amounts and becomes more sensitive. Concentrated urine can also irritate the bladder and the urethra. On the other hand, if you drink too much, you will have to urinate more often.

There are a number of reasons why people don't drink enough. The first has to do with habit. They have always drunk small amounts, perhaps because they have never been told why they should drink more. Or perhaps it is because they lead busy lives and don't always make the time to drink regularly during the day.

The second important reason people don't drink enough is more specific. If you have an irritable bladder and have problems with urgency and frequency, then it seems to make perfect sense to reduce these symptoms by drinking less. In the long term, however, this will serve to make the bladder more sensitive, not less.

How Much Should I Drink?

The recommended amount is around 3 pints (6 measuring cups) of liquid a day. It should be fairly easy for you to work out how much you usually drink. Count up the typical number of cups and glasses of whatever you drink in an average day and then measure how much this is by using water and a measuring cup. This will tell you whether or not you are drinking too much or too little. Obviously, the 3-pint rule is not a hard and fast one. It depends to a certain extent on your size and your level of activity. Also, in very hot climates, for example, it may be necessary to more than double this intake!

When Should I Drink It?

The answer is: regularly, throughout the day. It helps to get into a routine. Try to arrange it so that you are drinking a set amount every two hours. Of course, it makes sense to drink less in the evenings, beginning a couple of hours before bedtime, to avoid a disturbed night.

What Should I Drink?

If you have irritable bladder problems, it is important that you try to cut out caffeine. Caffeine is a stimulant and will increase the need to urinate. It is also a diuretic, which means that it encourages the kidneys to produce more urine.

Caffeine is found in coffee, tea and some soft drinks, such as colas. If the idea of giving them up fills you with total horror, then decaffeinated versions of these drinks are available. You can try phasing these alternatives in over time by, for example, alternating them with "the real thing" or making coffee or tea that is half and half. Over time, move over to having only the decaffeinated drinks. Some people are slightly addicted to caffeine, particularly if they drink more than eight cups of coffee a day. These people will notice withdrawal symptoms, such as headaches, if they try to cut down their intake too quickly.

The other thing to avoid (at least in excess) is alcohol. This, too, affects the bladder and is a diuretic. In fact, the dehydrating effect of alcohol is one of the main causes of the dreaded hangover.

Cranberry juice is thought to have beneficial effects on the bladder; otherwise the best thing to drink is water. Most of us are not used to drinking water on its own, mineral or otherwise, but it is possible to develop a taste for it. If the idea of drinking plain water appalls you, then watered-down fruit juice is a good alternative. Try to avoid too much straight fruit juice because it's too acidic and concentrated. In addition, a whole range of herbal teas is readily available, either by the bag or bottled, and these can be very refreshing.

Increasing Your Fluid Intake

As mentioned at the start of this chapter, the important thing is to go slowly. If you are worried about urgency and frequency, then increasing your fluid intake dramatically will demoralize you. If you think that you need to increase overall consumption by 1 pint a day, then that is about 2 cupfuls. Make it your goal to achieve this intake in a month's time. The first week of the month, have one extra drink in the middle of the day, each day. The second week, increase this to include an extra drink in the morning, and so on until you have reached your goal.

To motivate yourself, you could:

- ◆ Make a clear plan and write it down.
- ◆ Tell someone you are going to make this change.
- ◆ Keep a diary and check off your progress, reviewing it each week.
- ◆ Promise yourself a reward if you stick to your plan.
- ◆ Make a note of any benefits you notice.

Be aware that increasing your fluid intake over time may, in the short term, make the urgency and frequency seem worse, although most people find to their surprise that this doesn't happen. If you are particularly worried about increasing your fluid intake, make sure you begin when you can have a few days at home to see how you get along. Remember that focusing on the problem can make it worse, so it is important to keep yourself occupied.

In the long term, your bladder will learn to cope with holding more, particularly if you combine this with the advice in the next chapter. And remember, we are looking for benefits over weeks and months rather than days; it is important to change your habits slowly.

Decreasing Your Fluid Intake

Sometimes people drink too *much* out of habit. For example, it's easy to get into the habit of constantly putting the kettle on for a cup of tea or zapping an herbal tea bag in a mug of water in the microwave. Therefore, occasionally, problems of urgency and frequency are caused simply by drinking too much. If this is the case for you, keep a record of your intake and make a plan to monitor the number of drinks you have each day as described in the previous section, but instead of making it your goal to *increase* your intake over the next month, make it your goal to *decrease* it by the necessary amount.

Summary

Sometimes the fact that you are not drinking enough fluids can have long-term effects on your bladder. It is important to try to reverse these effects slowly. Certain kinds of drinks, such as coffee, tea and soft drinks, can adversely affect the bladder. Alcohol should also be avoided in excess, since it dehydrates the body.

CHAPTER SEVEN

Training Your Bladder

Bladder training is a very simple and successful way to overcome the problems of urgency, frequency and incontinence. In fact, it is the most commonly used and useful approach to combating them. Here I will describe how you can set up your own program. As in the last chapter, it is important to remember to make changes in a slow and steady manner if they are to be lasting. I will also describe how you can prepare for any setbacks. At the end of this chapter, I will describe pelvic floor exercises that can be either combined with bladder training or practiced separately.

What Is Bladder Training?

Bladder training is quite simply the process of getting your bladder to hold more urine for a longer period of time. You can train your bladder to do this by steadily increasing the time between visits to the toilet. Simple in theory, but not so simple in practice. To achieve this goal, what you need to be able to do is to resist the urge that you will inevitably feel to empty the bladder before you really need to. This is the essence of the problem, and the solution. If in the short term you can overcome the "false" messages from your bladder, eventually it will give up sending them. Your bladder will become less "irritable" over time. *You will be in control of your bladder;* your bladder will not control you.

Training your bladder involves the same principles as any other kind of training. Let's take the example of training a new puppy. We all know that if we want to encourage a dog to repeat a certain behavior, we reinforce it. If it sits when we tell it to sit, we give it a biscuit. Next time, the dog is more likely to sit when we tell it to sit because doing this has been linked with a pleasant thing. It is also possible to encourage "bad" behavior in a dog by reinforcing it without meaning to. Imagine that the dog barked when it was put out in the yard on its own. To stop the dog's barking, you let it in. This is a positive state of affairs for the dog; next time it is put out there it is more than likely to start barking again. If it is again let in you are "teaching" the dog that barking will cause it to be let in. You have unintentionally reinforced its barking behavior. If you are determined that your dog should get used to being outside, you will have to brace yourself to ignore the barking and only let it in after a set time or when it stops barking so that the "link" is unlearned.

Back to the bladder. The same principles apply. If your bladder starts sending strong messages to be emptied (the equivalent of the dog barking) and you respond immediately by going to the toilet (letting the dog in), you are encouraging your bladder to send even stronger urges under the same circumstances in the future. The positive state of affairs here is that you get *temporary* relief from the urgency and the worry associated with it. I stress the word temporary because in the long run you are encouraging the bladder to be more irritable, just as the dog was encouraged to bark. To stop your bladder "barking" at you, you need to brace yourself to tolerate the urges and empty your bladder only after a set time or when the urge has subsided. There are various things you can do to help yourself tolerate the urge, which I will discuss in more detail in Chapters 9 and 10, but that is the principle, and it works.

How Can I Train My Bladder?

The first step is to keep a diary noting the frequency, if you have not already done so. Note how often you are visiting the bathroom during the day. Most importantly, over a period of a few days, note what is the *longest* interval between visits to the bathroom that you have achieved? This is your starting point.

There won't be a typical figure, but what you *do* know is that your bladder can certainly go for whatever time the longest interval was without being emptied. What you will be doing, then, is setting an interval that you *know* you can achieve and emptying the bladder *only* at those times, ignoring urges to do so in between.

The best place to start is something slightly short of your "personal best" so that you know you can achieve it. If your diary shows that the longest you can hold on is an hour and 45 minutes, then you should choose to start at a set time of an hour and 30 minutes. Don't worry if you think your starting time should be an hour or even just 45 minutes—you need a goal that is a bit of a challenge, but not *too* daunting.

The very first day of your program will involve your only emptying the bladder when the set time is up, not earlier. Also, if you can hold on even longer, you should do so. It is a good idea not to rush to the bathroom the minute the time is up but to resist the first urge. Remember that you are trying to take control of these unwanted urges, so if you want them to go away you need to act as if they don't exist.

You can increase your set time by a few minutes each day if you want. However, this can be a bit confusing, and I suggest that you stick to each set time for two or three days, or even longer, until you are confident about that gap. Then increase the set time by 15 minutes. Again, do not go to the toilet until the time is up, and then resist the first urge after that and do not rush to the toilet. Continue to increase the gap by another 15 minutes once you are happy with that interval, and so on.

The program can take as long or short a period as you like. What you are aiming for is to be comfortable without emptying your bladder for three hours or more if you can. Some programs suggest going up to four hours, but I'm not sure many people *without* bladder problems do that. It is possible to increase the set time to three hours or more in just two weeks, but there is no *need* to go this fast. In fact, slow changes may be easier to stick to in the long run. These are the basic principles—you decide when to empty your bladder and you stick to it, despite messages to go earlier. You increase the amount of time between visits to the bathroom as you go along. Every time you ignore an unwanted urge, you are winning the battle.

At night, empty your bladder before going to bed, and then try to resist the urge to empty it within the next hour or so before you go to sleep. If you are in the habit of making "one last visit," even when you've just been, try the relaxation techniques described in Chapter 10 to get to sleep without doing this. If you wake up in the night and need to urinate, it is best to get up and do so, and then get right back to sleep. This ensures as little disturbance as possible. The efforts you make to control your bladder during the day will eventually pay off in terms of night-time urgency, without your having to make a special effort to tackle this problem.

Hints for Success

SUPPORT

When you are trying to make changes in your life, it is always much easier to achieve them if you feel supported. It helps if one or two trusted people know what you are trying to do so that they can support and encourage you. I hope you have managed to approach someone who can help.

It is also extremely important to support yourself by:

- Focusing on your successes, not your failures.
- Being patient and realistic about making changes.
- Not blaming yourself for your difficulties.
- Rewarding yourself.

PLANNING

The clearer you make your plans, the more likely you are to carry them out and achieve your goals. I have not given specific advice on things such as how often to empty the bladder, because everyone will need to start from a point that is appropriate to their own circumstances. However, this does not mean that you should not be specific with yourself—that is very important.

Planning and preparation often make all the difference to the success of a venture. Begin only when you are ready. Keep a diary to assess where you need to begin. Buy a special diary or notebook for the sole purpose of your program, and write on the first page some things you would like to achieve, such as going to the movies or starting an adult education or career advancement course. Write down this week's "personal best" and the set time you have decided on for the first few days of your program. Continue to keep the diary daily throughout your program, and write down your best time each week. Keep your supporter informed of any progress or difficulties.

To give the program the best chance of success, you may want to focus on it in the first week or two. This may mean taking a few days off work, or at the very least organizing things so that there is nothing to prevent you from sticking to the program. Of course, for it to work in the long term you will need to incorporate the principles of bladder training into your everyday life.

Plan some small goals into your program as well as the long-term goal. For example, if your overall goal is to achieve an interval of three and a half hours, plan a special prize for when you achieve a two-hour gap, a two-and-a-half-hour gap and so on. These can be whatever you like as long as you really like it! For example, a special treat might be to buy yourself something or watch a favorite video. I am sure you can think of things that will motivate you, but if you do find it difficult to come up with ideas it may be that you have gotten out of the habit of treating yourself. This is actually a very important source of motivation; make a list of activities that you have enjoyed in the past, or those that you have wanted to try; doing this should get the ideas flowing.

Do not begin the program until you have carefully planned what it will involve in practical and emotional terms. You may need to consider two more things before you begin. First, if you are worried about resisting the urge to urinate when it arises, it will help to practice relaxation and distraction techniques before you begin (see

Chapter 10). In addition, tensing the pelvic floor muscles can reduce the urge to urinate, so try the exercises at the end of this chapter. Remember that the more attention you focus on the bladder, the more sensations you are likely to notice. So, plan to keep busy and occupied, particularly if you are usually at work and decide to begin the program at home.

Second, you need to consider whether or not you have been avoiding a number of activities because of your bladder problems. It is often the case that people are able to keep to their program at home, but have difficulty at other times. This may be linked to worry. For example, going out shopping or traveling may be a worry because of your uncertainty about the restrooms available. This then leads to worries about your bladder, which can lead to increased sensations, which can lead to your making frequent visits to the bathroom before leaving home. You need to be particularly careful at these times and may need to anticipate these problems so that you can avoid them. Perhaps you may even decide to tackle such situations directly. When you have had some success with the training program, you can set a specific target, such as going to a certain shopping mall where you have already located and perhaps inspected the restrooms, and at the same time sticking to the program.

SETBACKS

Setbacks are *not* setbacks, they are learning experiences! There is always a reason for a setback, and it will teach you something about how to make more progress. Therefore, do not be afraid of setbacks.

Here are some common reasons for their occurring.

• *You have difficulty sticking to the program right from the start.* You may have set your sights too high. Remember, slow and steady; set yourself achievable targets. Or perhaps you just cannot fit the program into your lifestyle. In this case, be flexible. Remember that the principles of the program are to resist unwanted urges to urinate and to increase the time between visits to the bathroom these can be worked into any lifestyle. Try to wait for five extra minutes before emptying the bladder, or do one more small job before you go. Keep a record of the time between trips and try to improve on your personal best each week. If you apply these concepts, over time your symptoms will improve.

• *Something unexpected happens, something out of your control.* For example, you lose your job or someone in the family becomes ill. At such times you do not have the resources to stay with the program, and if the stress is great the problem may be as bad as ever. Cope as best you can and return to the program when things are more predictable.

• *You make good progress at home, but the symptoms return whenever you go away from home.* You need to do two things. First, acknowledge your fears about leaving the safety of home. If your fears have to do with trusting your bladder while you are out, you need to plan an additional program: increase the time and distance you can stay away from home. Practicing relaxation and challenging your fears will also help. What I mean by challenging your fears is to talk to yourself in a calming way. If you have the anxiety-provoking thought that it would be terrible to get the urge to urinate while out and not be able to find a restroom, ask yourself "Is this really likely to happen?" Remind yourself of your bladder's ability to hold on for however long you have achieved.

• *You make some initial progress, but cannot keep to the program.* Occasionally bladder problems are linked to anxiety, but often the anxiety originally had nothing to do with the bladder. When this is the case, as you begin to deal with the bladder problem another problem may emerge. If it is a difficult problem, it can lead to recurring bladder symptoms. Perhaps I should give an example.

> Rachel had always been shy and relied on her mother for support and encouragement. At the age of 18 she began college. She found that she had to keep rushing to the bathroom. She began to worry about this and tried to cope by drinking less and emptying her bladder whenever she had the opportunity. She remembered an incident during elementary school when she had a slight "accident" and worried that this would happen again.

> Eventually she gave up college and sought help for her bladder problems. Rachel quickly took to the principles of bladder

training. However, she had to deal with the setback caused by the realization that the anxiety that had led to the bladder problem originally was about becoming independent and coping in novel social situations. She began to tackle this by joining an evening class and taking trips out alone during the day to increase her self-confidence.

• *You have great initial success, but slowly slip back into your old ways.* Keep another diary and analyze what you are doing. Often people get into the habit of going to the bathroom "just in case" when it is not necessary. For example, they empty their bladders before leaving home regardless of how recently they have been or where they are going. It is rare for shops, restaurants or other people's houses to be toilet-free zones. Always ask yourself whether this trip to the toilet is actually necessary. Do you really have a full bladder—or is this merely a habit? Start yourself on a new program if this seems appropriate.

Pelvic Floor Exercises

If you have been told or suspect that pelvic floor muscle weakness plays a part in your bladder problems, doing appropriate exercises may help. In fact, pelvic floor exercises may even benefit urgency problems. There are two reasons for this. First, there is some evidence that tensing the pelvic floor muscles can help reduce the sensation of urgency that can be a problem in irritable bladder. Second, there is also evidence that some bladder problems are linked to difficulties relaxing the pelvic floor muscles when urinating. Learning to tense and relax these muscles at the right time may help you cope with your bladder problems. Also, following these exercises can increase the circulation around the pelvic area and may help with bowel problems, such as constipation.

What Are the Pelvic Floor Muscles and What Do They Do?

The pelvic floor muscles act like a taut hammock holding the bladder and bowel in place. Firm pelvic floor muscles prevent incontinence. When you urinate they relax, and after you stop they tighten up again. Weak muscles, however, mean that you may leak urine when you exercise, cough, sneeze or laugh.

What causes this weakness? The muscles can sag as a result of childbirth, lack of exercise, persistent coughing or constipation, being overweight, prostate or other surgery, or aging. In all of these cases, for both men and women, pelvic floor exercises can strengthen the muscles so that they give the correct support again.

How Do I Exercise My Pelvic Floor Muscles?

Pelvic floor exercises (kegel exercises) can be very effective if they are practiced correctly and persistently. Probably the hardest part of the exercise is motivating yourself to do them and remembering to do them often enough and over a long enough period of time. It is likely that you will have to practice for several weeks to notice a big improvement. You will have to make these exercises part of your everyday routine if you want to get results. The exercises themselves are simple. Try the following:

• Sit comfortably in a firm chair, leaning slightly forward, with your knees a bit apart. Imagine you are actually trying to stop yourself from passing gas. You should feel the pelvic floor muscles tighten and lift, without moving your legs, buttocks or stomach muscles.

• This time, imagine you are stopping the stream of urine mid flow, and again you should feel the muscles lift.

• Do both these lifts together. You should feel the whole area tighten and lift; this is the effect you want.

• Practice tensing the pelvic floor muscles by tensing and pulling up the muscles slowly and holding them as tight as you can for five seconds, or as long as you can at first, and then relaxing them to a count of five. Repeat this process five times. Then, pull up and tense the muscles quickly and relax them immediately in five quick squeezes. That's it, five slow and five quick tenses. Repeat this exercise ten times a day.

You can actually try to stop your flow of urine next time you go to the bathroom, halfway through emptying your bladder, and then relaxing again. You may not be successful if the muscles are weak, but if you are then you know you are tensing the correct muscles when you do the exercises. This test should not be repeated too often because it is important that you always completely empty the bladder. Try it once a week to assess your progress.

SOME ADDITIONAL TIPS

Use tricks to remind yourself to do the exercises, such as doing them every hour, checking off each time you do them.

It helps to tense up the pelvic floor muscles before you sneeze or cough or if you are trying to resist the urge to urinate.

SOME ALTERNATIVES

If you have difficulty doing the exercises correctly or are not having any success, there are a number of other approaches.

Cone therapy   This is a fairly new approach for women that has had some good results. Exercise the pelvic floor twice a day for 15 minutes by inserting a cone-shaped weight into the vagina and use the pelvic floor muscles to keep it in place. As the strength of these muscles increases, you can increase the weight of the cone you use. A sort of pelvic-floor weight training! The advantage is that you don't have to keep remembering to repeat tensing exercises throughout the day.

Electrotherapy   This is a way of making the muscle contract using special equipment. Electrodes need to be carefully positioned so that an electric current causes the correct stimulation. This kind of treatment is usually carried out by physiotherapists and is done at a clinic. It also requires you to continue practicing tensing and relaxing the muscle at home. Its usefulness primarily lies in learning which muscles to contract.

Perineometer   This is a piece of equipment that simply gives women feedback about pressure in the vagina so that they can see whether the exercises are being performed correctly. Over time, it can also give a measure of improvement, which can be very encouraging. Again, this equipment is available only in clinics, and success still relies on the long-term correct exercising of the pelvic floor.

Summary

Bladder training involves teaching the bladder to tolerate larger amounts of urine for longer periods of time. To do this, you need to learn to ignore the urge to empty the bladder and to do so only after a set time. This set time should be increased gradually until you can last from three to four hours. The program is flexible and you should design one that's best for you. You may need to learn ways of resisting the urge to empty the bladder, such as relaxation and distraction techniques. Sometimes worries about the bladder or other life problems may need to be tackled before lasting progress can be made.

Strengthening and becoming aware of the pelvic floor muscles can help with bladder symptoms. To truly benefit from pelvic floor exercises, you need to practice them every day for several weeks. Other therapies can offer women an alternative approach to the tensing exercises.

CHAPTER EIGHT

Health and Relationships

In Chapter 4 I discussed a number of factors that can affect how the bladder works. I touched on the fact that the bladder can be influenced by your lifestyle, your diet and how much exercise you get. Such factors are often difficult to change, but you may have little chance of overcoming your bladder difficulties unless they are addressed. Just as the bladder is influenced by outside factors, so can these factors be influenced by bladder problems. For example, having bladder problems may lead to a restricted lifestyle, which may lead to a lack of exercise, which may lead to weight problems, which may affect the bladder, and so on. Just as you have designed a program of bladder training for yourself, you may need to tackle some of these other problems as well.

The other important area where bladder problems can have an effect is in your personal relationships. In general, relationships can be altered, but sexual relationships may be particularly difficult when it comes to dealing with bladder problems. This chapter is about both health and relationships.

Diet

We hear a lot about what we should and should not eat. Sometimes it seems as if *all* foods are bad for us! We are also bombarded with images of "perfect" bodies and stories of those whose lives were transformed by losing weight.

All of this information can sometimes make us to forget about our *own* body's needs. We are all different, and there is no ideal diet or weight; it varies according to age, genes, lifestyle and build. It is now widely accepted that very low-calorie diets are bad for you in the long run because your body slows down to conserve energy, and when you start to eat normal foods you gain weight again.

The bladder may be adversely affected by being overweight or by chronic constipation. If either of these are long-standing problems for you, it may help to seek some advice and support from your family physician. The doctor may refer you to a dietitian. Everyone can benefit from an improved diet; dietary changes can have quite a noticeable effect on mood and energy levels. Here are some important things to remember.

• Habits that you change slowly are more likely to be lasting changes. Crash diets are not the answer to obesity because you cannot be on them forever. You must be able to live the rest of your life with your eating habits.

• Be flexible. Allow yourself some indulgences. Listen to your body and give it what it needs. Eat small amounts regularly during the day rather than eating a lot at night when you don't need the energy. Make time to plan, prepare and eat meals rather than eating on the run.

• Many of us, particularly women, have problems distinguishing between hunger and emotional states, such as distress and anger. This is often learned at a very early age and can lead to problems of over- or undereating. Recognize if this applies to you and try to learn new ways of dealing with emotional situations.

• The best advice is to make sure you have enough fiber in your diet to prevent constipation (fruit, vegetables and high-fiber cereals) and to cut down on fats (cheese, cream, butter) and refined sugars (sweets, chocolate, cake) wherever possible. When you go shopping, take a list and stick to it, and don't buy high-fat and high-sugar content products. If they are not in the house, you are less likely to eat them!

◆ Occasionally cases of irritable bladder have been helped by a gluten-free diet. If you suspect that you have a food allergy, ask your doctor or holistic practitioner for advice and help.

◆ Foods that increase the acidity of your urine can irritate the bladder and may encourage infection, particularly in women. To avoid this, do not drink excessive quantities of alcohol, cut out caffeine, eat moderate amounts of citrus fruit or soft fruits like strawberries, and don't eat large quantities of spicy foods. You can reduce the acidity of your urine by drinking plenty of water.

Exercise

Many of us fail to exercise enough. This may be a result of our busy lifestyles, which leave us too exhausted mentally and lacking the time to exercise. Or it may be a result of a restricted lifestyle where exercise is avoided because of bladder worries.

Exercising regularly is important for your general health and disposition as well as a remedy for specific problems, such as weakened muscles. Exercise does not have to be tortuous to be beneficial. Do not let memories of physical education at school put you off. As with dietary changes, the main mistake that people make is to try to do too much too soon, only to end up discouraged. You are not aiming for the Olympics! The important thing is to make small but lasting changes.

Gentle exercise can be very relaxing and have a positive effect on your sense of well-being. There is no lifestyle that excludes all forms of exercise—you do not need to spend a fortune on expensive equipment and gym fees or miss your lunch hour trying to fit in a game of tennis. Walking is one of the best forms of exercise. Simply walking for ten minutes, three times a week, until you build up to half an hour three times a week will make a big difference. Make sure you allow yourself the time; enlist a companion or take a cassette player along with you.

If you have particular health problems that make it difficult to walk, it might be worth asking to see a physiotherapist for some advice. If you are worried about exercising because of your bladder problems, remember that the long-term effect of exercising, in terms of mood and muscle tone, will be beneficial, and you do not have to do particularly strenuous movements to keep fit. In fact, the walking program may kill two birds with one stone—increasing your fitness and overcoming your fear of being away from home for a period of time.

Hygiene and Clothing

There are some simple, effective tips women (in particular) can follow to avoid bladder infection and genital irritation.

• Shower regularly rather than bathe. Use gentle soaps rather than highly scented ones, since they can irritate your sensitive urogenital area. Don't use feminine deodorants or disinfectants, for the same reason.

• Avoid tight clothing. Tight jeans and other clothes put unwanted pressure on the bladder. Wear cotton underwear and avoid nylon tights, especially in summer, because the dampness they create encourages fungal infections.

• Always take the time to empty your bladder and bowels completely, without rushing.

• It is a good idea to empty your bladder before and after sex. If you have urgency or leakage problems, you are better able to relax with your partner because your bladder is empty. One of the main causes of bladder infection is bacteria being encouraged up the urethra during intercourse, but these are flushed out by emptying the bladder afterward, minimizing the chances of an infection's occurring. If you are particularly prone to infections, then showering or rinsing the genital area before and after sex as well is also advisable. This may all sound like a lot of effort, but those who have suffered the misery of bladder infections will know that *any* means of avoiding them is worth its weight in gold (to say nothing of saving you the cost of a few visits to the doctor)!

Intimate Relationships

Irritable bladder problems can affect your sexual relationships in a number of ways. We all know that worries and distractions of any kind can interfere with the enjoyment that you can achieve with your partner. This can lead to tension in a relationship that, if not resolved, can over time lead to further problems, such as an avoidance of intimate situations. You might worry that your partner thinks less of you because of the bladder problems, or you may be too focused on the bladder symptoms themselves.

Obviously, it can be difficult to bring up these worries with your partner. However, sometimes simply voicing your fears is all that is needed to clear the air and allow you to relax again. You can also put your relaxation techniques into practice and focus your attention on the pleasurable sensations rather than those coming from your bladder. Worrying about urgency only makes it worse.

If it has been hard for you to talk about sexual situations and you are completely avoiding sex, an open discussion and agreement about gradually experimenting with greater intimacy is probably the best step forward.

To ease your mind, before you engage in sex empty your bladder. If you are worried about incontinence, try putting a towel over the sheet and remember that urine is sterile and odorless when it leaves the body.

Some people have specific sexual difficulties that are either related to or were there prior to the bladder problem, such as impotence or premature ejaculation in men and vaginismus or difficulty reaching orgasm in women. These difficulties, too, are made worse by worry and anxiety, but they can be overcome given the appropriate help. Unfortunately, it is beyond the scope of this book to delve into these areas, but there are many good books and resources available if you think that this applies to you or your partner.

As with other aspects of bladder problems, bladder and sexual worries can be made worse by worry, and this worry is often about the problem itself, creating a vicious circle. Tackling the problem *and* the worry together is the best strategy. Sometimes, on the other hand, the worry that is adding to the problem is related to another aspect of your life. If you are feeling very stressed at work, you may have trouble relaxing in a sexual situation, which causes you to worry, which then adds to your difficulty relaxing in the next sexual situation, and so on. Sometimes the original stressful situation needs to be resolved. Is it possible that stress in one area of your life is affecting both your bladder and your relationships? Try to figure out what needs to be addressed.

It is not uncommon for a difficult relationship itself to be the major source of stress that is affecting your bladder and sexual problems. If your relationship is already strained, it will be difficult to overcome these. Again, try to figure out what needs to be worked on.

Sexual violence or physical abuse is very difficult to talk about and can remain a hidden trauma for many women and also men. Yet it has been a reality for large numbers of people at some stage in their lives. Obviously such experiences have wide-ranging influences on relationships and sexuality. If such experiences were a reality for you and you feel your relationships are affected by them, I would encourage you to find the appropriate help you need to recognize how to overcome this trauma. This may be a very hard step to take, but the only one that will take you forward.

Summary

Your bladder is influenced by your general health and emotional well-being. Sometimes there are steps you have to take to improve these, before your bladder problems can be overcome.

Slow and steady changes in diet and exercise will be easier to stick to and will bring long-term benefits.

Bladder worries can have an adverse effect on intimate relationships. Discussing these problems is often avoided because of embarrassment, but tackling the difficulty is the only lasting solution.

CHAPTER NINE

Stress and the Bladder

As we now know, the bladder is clearly influenced by stress, "nerves" and worry. This is true for everyone, but it can be a particular problem for some people. Stress leads to a feeling of urgency, which can trick you into thinking that you need to empty your bladder. Think of times you've visited the bathroom before an important event only to find that you didn't really need to go after all. Being nervous stimulated the bladder, so you worried about needing to urinate and rushed to try to relieve the feeling. When the "nerves" passed and the "big event" was over, you were usually no longer aware of the urgency feeling. Of course, if you are stressed much of the time or if it is the bladder problem itself that is stressing you, then this sense of urgency can become a longer-term problem.

What do we mean by stress? What are the signs of stress? How can you tell if stress is playing a part in your irritable bladder problems? And most importantly, what can be done to reduce stress?

What Is Stress?

Stress is one of those contemporary words that we hear so often we think we know what it means. The truth is there are many different ways of understanding and defining stress. Even psychologists who specialize in this area disagree about how best to define it.

For our purposes we will look at three ways of thinking about stress. The first is that things in the world are stressful or difficult and put pressure on us; stress is simply "out there." This is what people mean when they talk about "stressful life events." What events are stressful? They are events that involve a change of some kind, such as moving, a job promotion or having a baby. As you can see from these examples, the events do not have to be bad things to be stressful. Generally, the more changes you have to cope with at any one time and the less control you have over the changes, the more stressed you are likely to be. Another factor that can add to our stress level is an ongoing problem, such as financial worries or relationship difficulties. Social support can help us deal with the stress of coping with the changes that come with such life events and ongoing strains. Social support means having good-quality relationships with family, friends or colleagues that allow you to talk through your problems, get information and decide how best to handle situations. There is one problem with this way of looking at stress, however: the same stressful life events for *us* may not have the same effect on someone else. For example, you may find public speaking extremely stressful, while Suzanne may actually enjoy it and even go on to make a living at it.

The second way of looking at stress is to think about the signs it exhibits in a person. The effects of stress can be broken down into short-term and long-term effects. When a person is in some immediate danger, the alarm reaction—the "fight or flight" response—is automatically triggered. You know what this response feels like if you have ever had a near-miss on the road or a similar experience. In the long-term effect, stress can have more wide-ranging effects on how we feel, behave, and think and on how our bodies work. These are described in more detail later. The trouble with this second approach is that although we may be able to see what it is like to be stressed, we don't fully understand why stress happens—or know what to do about it.

Seeing stress as "out there" as in the first approach or "in here" as in the second approach does not get us very far.

The third way to think about stress is to join both these ideas together. As human beings we are constantly trying to solve problems and perform well in the world. Constant demands (either by ourselves or by others) are made on us and, up to a certain point, they help us achieve our goals, which makes us feel more confident. However, when we think that the demands placed on us are too great, we experience stress. The way that we cope in the face of such demands and how many demands we put on ourselves determines how stressed we are. The important point to remember is that stress is a very individual thing. There are no universal rules about stress because:

• *We put demands on ourselves.* Of course, the world is unpredictable and stressful life events happen, like losing a job or flunking the bar exam or someone close to us dying, but for the most part, we put demands on ourselves. For example, we say to ourselves we "should" work late, we "ought to"help others more, we "must" get that promotion. These are individual demands; they are a result of our perception of our role and purpose in life. These are a result of a complicated process of socialization.

• *We experience stress when we think that we cannot cope.* This means that, in the face of a problem, we might feel that we don't have the ability to manage emotionally or practically. We may feel this way because of the manner in which we have handled similar problems in the past or because we lack knowledge or support. However, if we can solve a problem, sidestep it or accept it, we do not experience stress.

What does all this have to do with your bladder problem? It is important in two ways. First, if you feel you are not coping with the demands placed on you, then you will feel stressed, which can worsen your bladder symptoms. Second, bladder problems themselves place a high demand on your ability to cope. This is made worse by the taboo around the subject. Many people do not have the information about their problem or the means to cope effectively with it because it is hard for them to talk about it. And since it is hard for them to talk about it, they feel unsupported. The bladder problem continues because it is hidden, and the stress remains because the problem is not solved.

Are You Stressed?

A certain amount of stress is a *good* thing—it can be motivating and invigorating. Indeed, some people seem to thrive in high-stress situations, such as writers who are strongly motivated by deadlines, or rock climbers or stunt pilots. However, stress can also be unpleasant. Here are some of the unpleasant effects of stress.

Physical Effects

◆ *Short term.*   Increased heart and breathing rates, dizziness, sweating, blushing, shakes, nausea, butterflies in the stomach, frequent urination, diarrhea.

◆ *Long term.*   All of the above symptoms, plus high blood pressure, chest pain, headaches, bladder and bowel problems.

How You Think

Problems of concentration, difficulty making decisions, worrying, being overly self-critical, irrational ideas, fearfulness.

What You Do

You avoid stressful situations, go out of your way to escape talking to people, drink and smoke too much, eat more (or less), become irritable with those around you, get insomnia, suffer lack of sexual desire.

How Can Stress Cause So Many Different Symptoms?

Imagine that someone has just thrown a hand grenade into the room where you are sitting. Knowing immediately that you are in danger, adrenaline pumps through your body. This creates the "fight or flight" response. Breathing increases and your heart beats faster to supply more oxygen to the muscles in your legs so that you can run away very fast. Blood is diverted from nonessential areas to your major muscles; this explains the butterflies sensation in your stomach, because digestion is not an immediate need! You are ready to spring into action and run away.

We all have this mechanism, and it is very important that we do so that we can get out of danger. Of course, most situations that we see as threatening in modern life cannot be solved by fighting or running away. For example, if you are in danger of losing your job and this is a threatening state of affairs for you, your body will react with the same fight or flight response. However, even though you cannot solve this problem by literally running or fighting, your body will react with this stress response—as long as you see the situation as threatening. The longer the problem goes on, the more it will affect your health and well-being.

People find different things stressful and also feel the effects of stress differently. Try to think about the situations that you find stressful. Do they have anything in common? Is it possible to say what it is that makes these situations stressful for you? Is there anything you could learn or do to reduce your fears? How do you feel when you are stressed? Which particular symptoms do you experience? Can you identify any links between stressful situations and irritable bladder symptoms?

We now know that we experience stress when we see danger or a threat of any kind. This does not have to be a physical threat; it could be a threat to your self-esteem or to your health. This is how bladder problems, particularly incontinence, can be stressful. Such problems are often experienced as a major threat to your self-esteem.

How to Tackle Stress

As we have discussed, unpleasant stress occurs when we think of a situation as threatening. The three ways of tackling stress are:

• *Take direct action that solves the problem.*   If you use the example of your job's being threatened, direct action might include trying to find another job. If you take your bladder problem as an example of a potential threat to your self-esteem and health, then direct action might include going to the doctor or following self-help advice. If there are too many demands on you in general: prioritize, give things up, lower your standards a bit, ask other people to help you, plan some time for yourself. We all need time to unwind if we are to function at our best. Make sure you take proper breaks during the day, and relax on your days off. The body is a complicated machine that needs regular care in order to function. You should try to have at least an hour to yourself each day to relax and do the things you enjoy. If this seems impossible, then you need to think about your lifestyle and what you are trying to achieve.

Sometimes choosing not to reduce the demands on yourself means *choosing to be stressed*. If you find it hard to say "No" to people, you may often find yourself overloaded. Women in particular often feel uncomfortable about putting themselves first. Unfortunately, the problem with always putting *others* first is that you end up feeling stressed and exhausted. Make it a goal to become more assertive— buy a book on the topic or join a local support group. Being able to talk through your problems is often an essential part of solving them and keeping them in perspective. Have you lost touch with old friends and work colleagues? How can you go about starting to build some social support for yourself?

• *Think as realistically as possible about the situation.*   Try to avoid making emotional responses to your problems before you have all the information you need in order to understand the difficulty. Just because a situation *feels* hopeless, this does not mean that it *is* hopeless. Catastrophizing ("This is a terrible situation") and self-blame ("It's all my fault that this has happened") are very demotivating and prevent you from looking for solutions. What is the worst thing that can happen—and is it that bad? What resources do you have or could you create to help yourself? You can turn your problems into opportunities for learning, growth and change. Ask yourself what good things could come out of this difficulty. People are more likely to think in negative terms about situations that all of us fear, such as embarrassment, loss of control or illness. It is not surprising that irritable bladder sufferers are worried about their symptoms—and it is all the more reason to be as objective as possible about the situation.

• *Learn ways of keeping calm.*   Learning to keep calm is a skill that takes a lot of practice to achieve. It involves recognizing signs of stress, learning to relax, and noticing and challenging the thinking that makes situations seem more stressful ("It would be awful if . . ." or "I would just die if . . ." and so forth). Some ways of relaxing and keeping calm are described in the next chapter.

The Stress of Bladder Problems

Naturally, many people are worried about their bladder problems. And we know stress can affect the bladder, so how can these worries be overcome? The first thing to do is to get as much information as you can about the problem (this might be from reading or talking to health care professionals). Find out what can be done to help you and what you can do for yourself. Talk through the problem with someone supportive, and follow the advice given in this book. Do not blame yourself for your difficulties; bladder problems are nothing to be ashamed of. Try to tackle difficult situations and changes in lifestyle one step at a time.

Summary

This chapter has outlined the essentials of understanding and managing stress. If you wish to find out more, there are plenty of books devoted to the subject, and they can be helpful. If you think you are having problems with anxiety, or panic attacks, causing you to avoid situations, then you should consider talking to your family doctor who may be able to put you in touch with a trained nurse, counselor or psychologist who can help you to look at your particular problems and overcome them.

CHAPTER TEN

Learning to Relax

The title of this chapter is so named because I wish to emphasize that the techniques described are helpful only if they are practiced a lot! Just as it would be impossible for me to wake up tomorrow morning as a concert pianist, so it would be impossible for anyone to instantly become a stress-free and relaxed person. This is especially the case if your levels of stress and tension have been building up over many years. However, once you have mastered the basic techniques, you can put them into practice in everyday life so that as time goes by you get better at keeping your stress under control. Why is it good to relax? How can you learn to relax? What other techniques can be useful? This chapter will tell you.

Why Relax?

When you are relaxed, you are in the opposite state, physically and mentally, than you are in when you are stressed. Physical sensations are pleasant: you breathe calmly, your heart beats more slowly, your blood pressure falls, your muscles are relaxed. The psychological effects are enjoyable: you feel an inner calm, your mind has pleasant thoughts and images, you think more rationally. Over time you may sleep better, feel less tired, get fewer headaches as well as general aches and pains—and, I assure you, fewer irritable bladder problems. In fact, a number of studies on the subject have found that relaxation is extremely useful in the treatment of bladder problems. I have seen this for myself with many patients who can link their symptoms to stress or find themselves tensing up all the time. Discomfort and worrying about a particular part of the body often leads you instinctively to protect it by tensing up the muscles around the area. This is why those suffering from irritable bladder often report aches and pains in the lower back, abdomen and legs. Learning to release that tension can reduce your discomfort and lessen your symptoms. Other important reasons for employing relaxation are that it is free and it has no unwanted side effects!

How to Relax

We all have activities that we find relaxing, such as having a long hot bath, reading a weepy novel or watching television. What these activities usually have in common is that we are relatively still, there are no demands made on us and our minds are occupied with something pleasant. These are the essentials of relaxation, and you can learn to use them any place, any time—with a bit of practice!

To begin with, read through the rest of this chapter. As I stated before, it is not easy to change habits, and if you make progress in gradual steps you are more likely to be successful than if you try to achieve your goals too quickly. The more planning and commitment you put into any change, the more likely you are to succeed.

You will get the most benefit from practicing relaxation if you set aside 30 minutes each day for regular sessions. I can imagine some of you gasping, thinking that is impossible. If this is the case, your first task will be to work out how you are going to find this time: after lunch, when you get home from work or just before bedtime? Furthermore, you need to ensure that you have a quiet, warm room where you will not be disturbed. Make sure that other people in the house know this is your time, take the phone off the hook and hang a "do not disturb" sign on the door! The other thing you need is a comfortable place to be where your head can be slightly supported; this can be on the bed, on an exercise pad on the floor (or on a soft rug) with a thin pillow to support your head, or in a comfortable armchair.

There are a number of different relaxation techniques, but they all have three parts in common. The first is calm breathing; you should always start a relaxation session by calm breathing. The second is concentrating on the muscle tension in your body and working to release it. The third is holding calming images in your mind.

The reason for each of these components is that they add up to relaxation. When we are stressed we often breathe poorly. Relaxed breathing can lead to an immediate feeling of well-being. Muscle tension is a key result of being stressed and leads to many other harmful effects; it is important to learn how to let it go. Finally, stress symptoms in the body are often triggered by how we are thinking about a situation: If your mind is full of stressful thoughts such as "I must do so and so or else . . .," "It is terrible/awful that . . .," "I'll never manage . . .," then your body responds with a stress reaction. If, however, your mind is full of pleasant thoughts and images such as a favorite memory, a beautiful scene or a pleasant fantasy or daydream, then your body responds by relaxing.

I am going to describe each of the three stages: breathing, relaxing away tension and thinking calm thoughts. Some people prefer different parts of this process, and you may find that you benefit particularly from one but not the others. Practice each part separately and then together, and see what works best for you.

Relaxation is becoming much more popular these days as people acknowledge its benefits for health and well-being. It is easy to buy relaxation audio tapes. They are widely available from bookstores, health food stores and by mail order. Following a tape is often a good way of ensuring that you set aside enough time to relax completely. Not all tapes are the same, though, and you may have to try a couple before you find the right one for you. Self-hypnosis tapes usually combine calm breathing and visualization, and some people benefit from this form of relaxation. Although calm breathing and muscle relaxation can be practiced almost anywhere, imagery and visualization should be practiced only as part of a complete relaxation session, when you are lying or sitting peacefully. Do *not* listen to relaxation tapes or self-hypnosis tapes or practice imagery while you are driving or operating machinery!

A Breathing Exercise

1. Sit or lie comfortably while fully supported. Place one or both hands lightly on your stomach, close your eyes and breathe through your nose. Breathe slowly and deeply. Your stomach should rise and fall as you breathe in and out. This breathing should come naturally and not be an effort.

2. As you breathe in, feel your stomach rising; as you breathe out, say the word "calm" yourself. As you breathe out, breathe any tension away and allow your body to relax.

You should feel more relaxed, heavier and calmer. Practicing this for ten minutes a day can lead to an increased feeling of calm.

Relaxing Away Muscle Tension

Some people find that the breathing exercise is enough to relax their bodies and muscles completely, but if your body is very tense or there are specific areas of muscle tension, they may need direct attention.

Muscles will relax more if they are tensed up first and then relaxed, and this can be repeated to improve results. The process of tensing and relaxing also directs your attention to the muscular effects of stress; you may then recognize it's happening as you go about your everyday life, which allows you to release it before it builds up.

Some people find it useful to go through the whole body, tensing and relaxing the major muscle groups as part of their relaxation procedure. Others may choose to focus on a selection of specific muscles. The muscle groups most affected by tension are those in the neck and shoulders.

1. Sit or lie comfortably with your hands by your sides and your legs slightly apart. Close your eyes.

2. Take a deep breath in and breathe out slowly, saying the word "calm" to yourself as you do so. Keep breathing slowly and regularly throughout.

3. For each muscle group given below, inhale, tense those muscles for a count of five, and then breathe out and relax them. Focus on the relaxed muscles and then repeat once. The sequence for tensing the muscles is as follows:

- Make a tight fist with the hand you write with.

- Repeat using the other hand.

- To release tension in the upper arm, press your elbow back into the chair or bed or rug.

- Repeat using the other upper arm.

- To release tension in your face, clench your jaw, wrinkle your nose and wrinkle your forehead, as if you are trying to squeeze your eyes, nose and mouth into a tiny space.

- To release tension in your neck, press your head back against the chair or into the pillow.

- To release tension in your shoulders and chest, take a deep breath, push your chest out and your shoulders back.

- To release tension in your stomach, pull your muscles in.

- To release tension in your thighs, tense them up, and, if you are sitting, press your heels into the floor.

- To release tension in your calves and feet, point your toes away from your body and then curl them down.

When you have completed this sequence, focus for a few minutes on how the relaxed muscles feel and the overall sense of calm you feel.

This sequence is easier to follow while listening to a tape you have recorded because you don't have to think about what to do next. If you have any difficulty tensing and relaxing any muscle group or experience any pain, then leave them out of the sequence and concentrate on the breathing and visualization exercises.

A Visualization Exercise

When you have learned to feel relaxed using breathing techniques and muscle relaxation, then move on to visualization.

Choose a calm scene, either one from memory or one you can imagine. It could be anything; the most important thing is that you find it relaxing. For example, you might like to visualize yourself on a beach, curled up by a log fire or in the country. You should use all your senses to get absorbed in the scene, thinking about what you can see (colors, people, movement), hear (birds, water, wind, voices), touch (textures, temperatures) and smell (flowers, the sea).

1. Begin in the same position as the last two exercises, sitting or lying comfortably, closing your eyes and focusing on calm breathing. As you breathe out, say the word "calm" to yourself.

2. Begin to imagine in your mind's eye the scene you have chosen. Try to imagine as much detail as you can, as if you were actually there. If your mind drifts away from it, gently bring yourself back to the scene. It can take a lot of practice to keep your mind focused. Continue visualizing the scene for about ten minutes.

Some Hints

These three ways of relaxing—calm breathing, muscle relaxation and visualization—can be practiced separately or together as if in an exercise regimen. Keep practicing until you find which works best for you, and then practice your chosen exercise(s) regularly. Allow yourself time to relax completely, and get up slowly at the end of a session, after taking a couple of deep breaths.

Put the principles into practice in real life. If you feel yourself tensing up, relax the tension away (particularly when it occurs in the neck and shoulders), by breathing calmly and repeating the word "calm" to yourself as you breathe out. Ten minutes spent on these techniques in the middle of a hectic day can have quite an impact on your stress levels.

Relaxation and Irritable Bladder

Learning to relax will help you cope with your bladder symptoms and may directly improve them. Some people may have fears about relaxing and letting go, especially if they have been tense for a long time or they believe that the tension is protecting them in some way. If you have fears of incontinence, it is likely that you instinctively tense up your pelvic floor muscles, buttocks and stomach. Try a gradual program of tensing and relaxing these muscle groups, and remember to relax them if you feel yourself tensing up during the day. If you have weak pelvic floor muscles, you should consciously tense up the area before coughing, sneezing, laughing or lifting and then relax them again afterward. Sometimes, squeezing your pelvic floor muscles can help you resist the urge caused by an unwanted bladder contraction.

If you are training your bladder and trying to ignore the urge to urinate, then relaxation can help you with this. Focus on breathing and relaxation as a distraction from the sensations, repeating the word "calm" to yourself. Practice the visualization exercise, too, and use this for five or ten minutes when you want to delay emptying your bladder. Remember that if you focus on the discomfort, then it feels worse. Here are some distraction techniques.

Distraction Techniques

◆ *Focus on the world around you.*   Look at things surrounding you in great detail.

◆ *Focus on a particular object.*   Choose an object that conjures up happy associations, such as a photograph or souvenir. Focus on it and use it as a link into pleasant thoughts and memories.

◆ *Mind games.*   Do a short crossword puzzle, recite poetry, think of a boy's and a girl's name for each letter of the alphabet, listen to a language tape and try to learn new phrases—anything that takes your mind off your bladder.

◆ *Action.*   Go for a short walk, do a household chore, bake a cake, write a letter. Make a list of the activities you enjoy to refer to when you need to be distracted.

The principle behind such strategies is that it will be easier for you to resist unwanted bladder urges, making yourself and your bodily responses calmer in the future. Distracting your attention from your bladder using any of the above ideas—or whatever works best for you—will enable you to achieve this end.

Summary

Relaxation can be extremely beneficial in dealing with bladder problems. To get the maximum benefit, make it part of your daily routine, and put it into practice in stressful situations.

Relaxation involves calm breathing, relaxing muscle tension and focusing thoughts on a pleasant scene. These techniques and other ways of distracting your attention can be helpful in bladder retraining because they allow you to resist the urge to empty the bladder.

A Few Final Words

I hope that you have found the advice in this book helpful. Irritable bladder problems are much more common than you would expect and can develop for a number of reasons. The key points made in the book are summarized below. I wish you every success in coping with your irritable bladder.

Be aware of your symptoms.

Liquids—drink plenty of liquids and avoid caffeine.

Attitude—think positive.

Delay bladder emptying.

Distraction techniques—use them to draw attention away from your bladder.

Exercise the pelvic floor muscles.

Relax!

Relationships are important for support.

Unfulfilled ambitions need to be taken care of—fulfill them.

Lifestyle—think "diet, hygiene and fitness."

Expect to fail sometimes, it's okay.

Stress management.

Glossary of Medical Terms

Abdomen: The stomach area.

Anus: The opening of the bowel in your buttocks, which is controlled by sphincter muscles.

Bladder training: A program to increase the time gap between trips to the restroom to improve bladder capacity.

Cystitis: An infection of the bladder.

Cystoscopy: A visual examination of the inside of the bladder by means of a tiny camera passed up the urethra, performed under general or local anesthetic.

Diuretic: A substance that encourages the production of urine.

Hysterectomy: The surgical removal of the uterus.

Incontinence: Involuntary loss of urine.

Menopause: Hormonal changes in women, usually between the ages of 45 and 55, when menstrual periods cease.

Prolapse: Descent of the pelvic organs due to a weakening of the supporting muscles.

Prostate: A gland in men that surrounds the urethra just below the bladder neck; it produces fluid for semen.

Sphincter: A circular band of muscle that regulates the passage of fluids or solids through a tube.

Unstable bladder: A bladder that contracts on filling, causing a sudden and urgent desire to urinate.

Ureters: Thin tubes that run from the kidneys to the bladder.

Urethra: The two-inch tube leading from the bladder to the outside, in females and running through the penis in males.

Urodynamics: Tests to study the behavior of the bladder on filling and emptying.

Useful Addresses

National Association for Continence (NAFC)
P.O. Box 8310
Spartanburg, SC 29305-8310
   www.nafc.org
   800-BLADDER (252-3337), 864-579-7900
   fax 864-579-7902

Incontinence Control Clinic
   415-456-5699

Interstitial Cystitis Association (ICA)
P.O. Box 1553
Madison Square Station
New York, NY 10159
   info@aol.com,
   www.ichelp.com
   800-HELP-ICA (435-7422), 212-979-6057

Interstitial Cystitis Network
4773 Sonoma Highway #125
Santa Rosa, CA 95409
   www.sonic.net/jill/icnet
   707-538-9442
   fax 707-538-9444

Further Reading

CYSTITIS

Chalker, Rebecca, et al. *Overcoming Bladder Disorders*. HarperCollins, 1991.

Gillespie, Larrian and Sandra Blakeslee. *You Don't Have to Live with Cystitis*. Avon Books, 1996.

Kilmartin, Angela. *Understanding Cystitis: A Complete Self-Help Guide to Overcoming Thrush and Cystitis*. Arrow Books, 1989.

Newman, Diane Kaschak and Mary Dzurinko. *Urinary Incontinence Sourcebook*. Lowell House, 1997.

Young, Jacqueline. *Cystitis*. Element, 1997.

ASSERTIVENESS

Gutmann, Joanna. *The Assertiveness Workbook*. Sheldon, 1993.

Smith, Manuel. *When I Say No I Feel Guilty*. Bantam Books, 1981.

GENERAL

Burns, David. *Feeling Good: The New Mood Therapy*. Avon Books, 1992.

Index

NOTES

NOTES

ULYSSES PRESS HEALTH BOOKS

DISCOVER HANDBOOKS

Easy to follow and authoritative, *Discover Handbooks* reveal an array of alternative therapies from around the world and demonstrate how to incorporate them into a program of good health.

Each book opens with information on the history and principles of the particular technique, then presents practical and straightforward guidance on ways in which it can be applied. Offering the tools needed to achieve and maintain an optimal state of health, the approach is one of personal improvement and self-reliance. Each of the books features: an introduction to the discipline; an explanation of its philosophy; step-by-step guide to its implementation; clear diagrams and charts; and case studies.

DISCOVER AYURVEDA
ISBN 1-56975-081-5, 128 pp, $8.95

DISCOVER COLOR THERAPY
ISBN 1-56975-093-9, 144 pp, $8.95

DISCOVER ESSENTIAL OILS
ISBN 1-56975-080-7, 128 pp, $8.95

DISCOVER FLOWER ESSENCES
ISBN 1-56975-099-8, 120 pp, $8.95

DISCOVER MEDITATION
ISBN 1-56975-113-7, 144 pp, $8.95

DISCOVER NUTRITIONAL THERAPY
ISBN 1-56975-135-8, 120 pp, $8.95

DISCOVER OSTEOPATHY
ISBN 1-56975-115-3, 132 pp, $8.95

DISCOVER REFLEXOLOGY
ISBN 1-56975-112-9, 132 pp, $8.95

DISCOVER SHIATSU
ISBN 1-56975-082-3, 128 pp, $8.95

A Natural Approach Books

Written in a friendly, nontechnical style, *A Natural Approach* books address specific health issues and show you how to take an active part in your own treatment. Whether you suffer from panic attacks, endometriosis or depression, each book will provide you with a thorough understanding of your condition and detail organic solutions that offer immediate relief for your symptoms and effectively remedy their underlying causes.

Believing that disease is more than a combination of symptoms, these books offer integrated mind/body programs that take a positive, preventative approach. Since traditional drug therapy is not always the best solution (and can sometimes be the problem), these guides show how to use alternative treatments to supplement or replace conventional medicine.

ANXIETY & DEPRESSION
ISBN 1-56975-118-8, 144 pp, $9.95

ENDOMETRIOSIS
ISBN 1-56975-088-2, 120 pp, $8.95

FREE YOURSELF FROM TRANQUILIZERS
& SLEEPING PILLS
ISBN 1-56975-074-2, 192 pp, $9.95

IRRITABLE BLADDER & INCONTINENCE
ISBN 1-56975-089-0, 108 pp, $8.95

IRRITABLE BOWEL SYNDROME
ISBN 1-56975-030-0, 240 pp, $11.95

MIGRAINES
ISBN 1-56975-140-4, 156 pp, $8.95

PANIC ATTACKS
ISBN 1-56975-045-9, 148 pp, $8.95

The Natural Healer Books

As home remedies and alternative treatments become increasingly accepted into the medical mainstream, people want information—not just hype and unproven claims—about the remedies they see in health food stores. *The Natural Healer* books detail how these natural remedies have been used throughout history and how to safely incorporate them into an overall plan for maintaining good health.

CIDER VINEGAR
ISBN 1-56975-141-2, 120 pp, $8.95

GARLIC
ISBN 1-56975-097-1, 120 pp, $8.95

The Ancient and Healing Arts Books

The Ancient and Healing Arts books recount the development of healing art forms that have been used for thousands of years. Beautifully illustrated with full color on every page, they discuss the benefits of these time-honored techniques and offer detailed instructions on their use.

The Ancient and Healing Art of Aromatherapy
ISBN 1-56975-094-7, 96 pp, $14.95

The Ancient and Healing Art of Chinese Herbalism
ISBN 1-56975-139-0, 96 pp, $14.95

Other Health Titles

The Book of Kombucha
ISBN 1-56975-049-1, 160 pp, $11.95
Explains the benefits of and addresses concerns about Kombucha, the widely used Chinese "tea mushroom."

Hepatitis C: A Personal Guide to Good Health
ISBN 1-56975-091-2, 172 pp, $12.95
Identifies the causes and symptoms of hepatitis C and presents conventional and alternative treatments for coping with the disease.

Know Your Body: The Atlas of Anatomy
ISBN 1-56975-021-1, 160 pp, $12.95
Presents a full-color guide to the structure of the human body.

Mood Foods
ISBN 1-56975-023-8, 192 pp, $9.95
Shows how the foods you eat influence your emotions and behavior.

Your Natural Pregnancy: A Guide to Complementary Therapies
ISBN 1-56975-059-9, 240 pp, $16.95
Details alternative therapies ranging from aromatherapy to yoga that can benefit pregnant women.

To order these books call 800-377-2542, fax 510-601-8307 or write to Ulysses Press, P.O. Box 3440, Berkeley, CA 94703-3440. All retail orders are shipped free of charge. California residents must include sales tax. Allow two to three weeks for delivery.

Dr. Jennifer Hunt specializes in health psychology and has published a number of articles on bladder problems.